# Trauma, Survival and Resilience in War Zones

This book, based upon a series of psychological research studies, examines Sierra Leone as a case study of a constructivist and narrative perspective on psychological responses to warfare, telling the stories of a range of survivors of the civil war. The authors explore previous research on psychological responses to warfare while providing background information on the Sierra Leone civil war and its context.

Chapters consider particular groups of survivors, including former child soldiers, as well as amputee footballers, mental health service users and providers, and refugees. Implications of the themes emerging from this research are considered with respect to how new understandings can inform current models of trauma and work with its survivors. Amongst the issues concerned will be post-traumatic stress and post-traumatic growth; resilience; mental health service provision; perpetration of atrocities; and forgiveness. The book also provides a critical consideration of the appropriateness of the use of Western concepts and methods in an African context.

Drawing upon psychological theory and rich narrative research, *Trauma, Survival and Resilience in War Zones* will appeal to researchers and academics in the field of clinical psychology, as well as those studying post-war conflict zones.

**David A. Winter** is Professor of Clinical Psychology and Programme Director of the Doctorate in Clinical Psychology at the University of Hertfordshire, UK. During the completion of this book, he was also Visiting Professor in the Department of General Psychology at the University of Padua, Italy.

**Rachel Brown** completed her Doctorate in Clinical Psychology at the University of Hertfordshire, UK, in 2013.

**Stephanie Goins** serves as Executive Programs Director for Love146, a non-profit organization that works to abolish child exploitation and trafficking.

**Clare Mason** completed a Master's in Psychology at the University of Hertfordshire, UK, in 2013.

# Explorations in Mental Health Series

Books in this series:

# Trauma, Survival and Resilience in War Zones

The psychological impact of war in Sierra Leone and beyond

David A. Winter, Rachel Brown, Stephanie Goins and Clare Mason

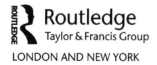

Routledge
Taylor & Francis Group

LONDON AND NEW YORK

First published 2016 by Routledge

2 Park Square, Milton Park, Abingdon, Oxfordshire OX14 4RN
711 Third Avenue, New York, NY 10017

*Routledge is an imprint of the Taylor & Francis Group,
an informa business*

First issued in paperback 2017

*British Library Cataloguing in Publication Data*
A catalogue record for this book is available from the British
Library

*Library of Congress Cataloging-in-Publication Data*
Winter, David A., 1950–
    Trauma, survival and resilience in war zones : the psychological
impact of war in Sierra Leone and beyond / David A. Winter,
Rachel Brown, Stephanie Goins and Clare Mason.
        pages cm
    Includes bibliographical references and index.
    1. War victims—Mental health—Sierra Leone.   2. Post-traumatic
stress disorder—Sierra Leone.   3. Resilience (Personality trait)—
Sierra Leone.   4. Children and war—Sierra Leone—Psychological
aspects.   I. Brown, Rachel (Psychologist)   II. Goins, Stephanie.
III. Mason, Clare.   IV. Title.
    RC550.W56  2016
    616.85′21009664—dc23
    2015020092

ISBN: 978-1-138-79969-1 (hbk)
ISBN: 978-0-8153-5890-9 (pbk)


Typeset in Bembo
by Apex CoVantage, LLC

# Contents

**PART 3**
# Implications                                                  153

*Asking questions will enable one to find the right answer.*
Mende proverb

# Preface

The West African country of Sierra Leone is a land of marked contrasts. Its Muslim and Christian communities live in harmony, but it has experienced eleven years of brutal civil war. It has breathtaking beauty and natural resources, but these, in the form of 'blood diamonds', have brought not wealth but terror and poverty to many of its population. Its children have heart-warming smiles, but have been both victims and perpetrators of unimaginable horror. Its capital, Freetown, was a home for freed slaves, but those of its citizens who express themselves in ways which do not fit in with dominant societal ideals may find themselves kept in chains.

This book has arisen from each of us having been profoundly affected by our encounters with survivors of Sierra Leone's civil war in the course of research, teaching, clinical practice and/or friendship. We have been particularly struck by the resilience of the people of a country that seems to have had much more than its fair share of tribulation and that, as we have been writing the book, has been undergoing yet more suffering due to the Ebola epidemic. In the following pages, we shall attempt to do justice to, and learn from, the stories of these extraordinary people. Based on a series of psychological research studies, Sierra Leone will be used as a case study of a constructivist and narrative perspective on psychological responses to warfare.

The first section of the book will provide a background to previous theoretical perspectives and research on psychological responses to warfare, as well as to the people of Sierra Leone and the civil war that ravaged their country and its context. In the second section, we shall present the stories of a range of survivors of the war, including former child soldiers, amputee footballers, mental health service users and providers, and refugees. These individuals' stories will be told largely in their own words, using data gathered with a range of qualitative and quantitative research methods. In the final section, implications of the themes emerging from these stories will be considered with respect to how new understandings can inform current models of trauma and work with its survivors. Amongst the issues concerned will be post-traumatic stress and post-traumatic growth, resilience, mental health service provision, perpetration of atrocities and forgiveness. There will also be critical consideration of the appropriateness of the use of Western concepts and methods in an African context.

We are enormously indebted to the people of Sierra Leone who willingly and generously shared their stories with us. It is impossible for us to mention all of those who have contributed in one way or another to the work reported in this book, but we each wish to make a few particular acknowledgements, and to apologize to those whom we have failed to include, and in several cases whose names we do not know. These acknowledgements are as follows.

David: I wish to express my gratitude to Aneurin Braimah, Susan Bridi, Dr Sulaiman Kabba, Funmi Ladeinde, Dr Sarah Maclean, Dr Edward Nahim, Dr Louise Scrivener, Dr Josefin Sundin, Silvia Urbano Giralt, Heleen van den Brink, Dr Nick Wood, the Sierra Leone Single-Leg Amputee Football Club and other amputee footballers who contributed to the research, and to fellow members of the Barnet, Enfield and Haringey Sierra Leone Project Implementation Group, in particular Dr Ros Furlong, Dr Denny Grant and Norma Johnson. I also wish to thank my coauthors for agreeing so readily to join me in this venture, and for doing so with such dedication.

Rachel: I was privileged to have heard the stories told within this research, and I wish to acknowledge the participants who allowed me to step momentarily into their lives; I have been irrevocably changed by their stories. I would also like to acknowledge the contributions of Dr Saskia Keville and Dr Nick Wood, who played a key role in supervising, alongside Professor David Winter, the research described in Chapter 8. I also wish to offer my heartfelt thanks to Aminata Mansaray and Sarah Jones for patiently sharing with me their experience and local knowledge of Sierra Leone.

Stephanie: The people of Sierra Leone won my heart and my admiration with their welcome, their warmth and their resilience. I am particularly grateful for my translator, who provided tremendous insight into the psyche of Sierra Leone people and the challenges they faced with post-war recovery. I want to thank my husband, J., who has always been supportive of my passion and work. And last, I would like to thank Dr David Winter, who convinced me that my work in Sierra Leone was a story that should be told.

Clare: I would like to express my heartfelt thanks to the survivors of the Sierra Leone civil war whom I met during the course of this book. Their generosity in sharing personal and often painful stories, and their ability to rebuild troubled lives, remains an inspiration. I would also like to thank Professor David Winter for the opportunity to develop further this area of interest. Finally, warmest thanks must go to my children, Laura, James and Julia, for being the most wonderful of distractions throughout.

# Part 1

# Background

# Chapter 1

# A typical encounter in Freetown

One of us (David) was walking to his hotel in Freetown one Sunday when he was greeted with a shout of 'How de body?'[1] by a very smartly dressed man wearing a suit and the extravagant shoes (in this case, perhaps made of crocodile skin) that are popular in Sierra Leone. David returned the greeting ('De body fine!'[2]), and then did a 'double take' as he became aware that the man looked familiar. The realization then dawned that he was someone, whom we shall call Samuel, who on every one of David's six visits to Freetown had always magically appeared on his first or second day in town, wherever he might be, and had asked to be hired as his 'minder'. Reminders of the legacy of the civil war were never far away in Freetown and its outskirts: occasional skirmishes between opposing political factions; graffiti advertising gangs with names such as Blade Squad, Murder Inc., One Shot Squad, Black Sword, and Terror Squad; and makeshift roadblocks manned (or 'boyed') by youths demanding money, through which one would drive without stopping if one were feeling brave enough. Despite these, and despite the pitch-blackness of the nights, unlit by electricity, David rarely felt any more need of a minder in Freetown than in the English village in which he lives. Nevertheless, he used to give Samuel a few thousand leones[3] (and a Star beer on the occasions when he would again suddenly appear in any bar where David happened to be trying to have a quiet drink after a long, hard day) to be his official minder, largely in order to obtain some relief from Samuel's constant insistence on David's need for such protection and his own need for the money with which this would provide him.

While, to be honest, David generally found Samuel's chatter tiresome and tried to avoid him, this Sunday was different, as David was curious about the dramatic change in his appearance from the rather disreputable-looking character with whom he was more familiar. David therefore asked why he was dressed so well, and he said that he did this every Sunday in order to go to church and obtain forgiveness from God for what he had done in the war. David's curiosity was further aroused, and they agreed to continue the conversation the next day. It went like this:

*Samuel:* The war normally it has affected many Sierra Leoneans. And then the ones like me they forced me to fight in the war. And then when when

I'm fighting the war I do much killing and then the rebels, Kamajor,[4] and then the rebels and the SLA[5] and . . . then they're killing each other and then by the end they asked us to come together and then finish with the war. By then there was big trouble . . . because there was more more, more killing more, more, more catastrophe many, many, many problems in Sierra Leone people don't have nothing to eat, people are eating dogs, many people to be crazy, locked up, getting mad, many, many.

David:    How old were you when they forced you to fight?

Samuel:   I was just 11, 12 years and a half.

David:    What happened?

Samuel:   Well, they catch me in the village in a raid during the night the rebels and then they catch the young girls and young boys; they say you must join us and then they forced them into sexual abuse the ladies, the young girls, take them to the forest. They say if you don't go with us we kill you. And they give me gun, give my colleagues gun, basically we join them.

David:    And what did they force you to do?

Samuel:   They forced me to fire, they say to attack ECOMOG,[6] Nigerian soldiers, we must launch attack, we must fight against them, they are enemies.

David:    So you were using the gun when you were 12?

Samuel:   Yes, I was using the gun, they gave me the biggest gun to carry. I was a young boy and they forced me to shoot and I killed.

David:    How many did you kill?

Samuel:   Many, many people, maybe 50, maybe 100 people I killed. I saved my parents because when I fight none of them die but we suffered because we don't have nothing to eat.

David:    People who know you fought with the rebels, how do they feel about you now?

Samuel:   Normally now they think I've changed because I'm trying to get my family, I have my baby, and I get my wife, so they think I've changed and then I used to go to church because I want to be a godly man. I used to go to church every Sunday.

David:    During the war how, how did you feel about yourself?

Samuel:   During the war, because they give me drugs I was very nasty but now I appreciate the way I feel because I feel good and Sierra Leone is peaceful so we need help from the outside world to help us so Sierra Leone can be a good place.

Samuel's story encapsulates much of the experience of living in Sierra Leone, and in other countries in post-conflict situations. First, one never knows whether the affable façade with which one is presented conceals a darker past. Literally, one never knows whether the hand that one is shaking may have taken many lives (in the case of Samuel, probably more than the 50 to 100 to which he admitted) or inflicted unspeakable atrocities. Indeed, victims of such atrocities may find themselves in daily contact in their communities with the perpetrators of these.

Also apparent is some of the confusion that was experienced in a conflict in which various different groups (e.g. rebels, Kamajors, the SLA and ECOMOG) were killing each other, and in which some of this killing was done by children, who were often faced with a choice between killing and being killed. As in Samuel's case, a degree of self-esteem could be maintained by viewing one's actions as having been carried out under duress or the influence of drugs. His account also reveals a desire to move on to a more peaceful life, both for himself and his country, albeit, as is repeated again and again in the stories of war survivors, with a need for outside help. In addition, it indicates that others have been unable to show the same resilience but instead may find themselves locked up and 'crazy'.

All of these trajectories will be evident in the accounts that we shall present, but first we shall review the literature on the psychological effects of warfare and provide more of a background to the situation in Sierra Leone.

## Notes

1  How's the body?
2  The body's fine!
3  1 English pound = approximately 6,400 leones.
4  Originally secret society members, with supposed supernatural powers, who fought as a civil defence group in the civil war.
5  Sierra Leone Army.
6  Economic Community of West African States Monitoring Group.

# Chapter 2

# Psychological responses to warfare

Warfare has been taking place across the world for an inordinate number of years. Widespread death and injury inevitably result. For both combatants and civilians, war presents numerous traumatic experiences. Traumatic events can threaten an individual's perception of self and the world. Because much of psychology's knowledge of the impact of trauma stems from individuals seeking help, it has often been assumed that a pathological response is the most common. In reality, the majority of people are resilient to trauma and continue to live emotionally positive and fully functioning lives. This is not to underestimate the very severe difficulties of those who develop post-traumatic stress disorder; rather, it recognizes that not everyone reacts to trauma in the same way. Why some individuals demonstrate resilience, others progress to post-traumatic growth, whilst yet others are affected by post-traumatic stress disorder is a reflection of the heterogeneity and uniqueness of life experiences. It is, therefore, imperative to be sensitive to the cultural context of the individuals and situations concerned. This chapter provides an overview of relevant literature, highlighting the most salient issues concerning the psychological responses to warfare.

## Resilience in the face of trauma

Initial research into the psychology of traumatic events focused on psychopathological responses (Hobfoll, Mancini, Hall, Canetti & Bonanno, 2011). However, there is now overwhelming evidence that most people respond to trauma with minimal disruption to their overall functioning and, instead, demonstrate resilience (Bonanno, Westphal & Mancini, 2011). According to Masten (2011), resilience can be defined as the capacity to withstand or recover from significant challenges that threaten stability, viability or development. Bonanno, Westphal and Mancini (2011, p. 513) more specifically define it as 'an outcome pattern following a potentially traumatic event (PTE) characterized by a stable trajectory of healthy psychological and physical functioning'. Empirical data led Bonanno (2004) to propose that whilst there is a natural heterogeneity to the human response, most of this can be captured in a set of four prototypical outcomes. These have been found to be remarkably consistent across a number of studies (Bonanno, 2012):

*Prototypical trajectories of adjustment following a PTE (and relative prevalence) (Bonanno, 2004; Bonanno, Westphal & Mancini, 2011).*

(i) *Resilience (35–65%)*

> Resilience is typified by transient symptoms of minimum impairment followed, relatively soon after the PTE, by a stable trajectory of healthy functioning.

(ii) *Recovery (15–25%)*

> Recovery involves initial elevated symptoms with some functional impairment, followed by a gradual return to normal levels of functioning.

(iii) *Chronic Distress (Post-Traumatic Stress Disorder [PTSD]) (5–30%)*

> PTSD is characterized by a sharp elevation in symptoms and functional impairment that persist for a long time after the PTE.

(iv) *Delayed Distress (0–15%)*

> Delayed distress is distinguished by moderate to elevated symptoms soon after the PTE, with a gradual worsening over time.

For many years a resilient response to a PTE was considered atypical, a result of heightened emotional strength or the converse, a complete numbing of emotions. Indeed, the view of the absence of distress and dysfunction as an abnormal reaction continues to persist amongst many of the lay public. Nevertheless, as Masten (2001) maintains, the capacity for resilience lies well within the range of ordinary human capabilities.

Whilst recovery may be considered in alignment with resilience, Bonanno et al. (2011) emphasize a contrasting path. They maintain that individuals experiencing recovery will, by definition, have suffered a level of acute distress before returning to normal functioning. In contrast, resilience is characterized by a minor and transient level of distress, with minimal function disruption.

### Factors affecting resilience

As resilience is the prevailing response to a PTE, consideration of influencing factors must reflect the heterogeneity of the individuals and circumstances involved. In their investigation of the roles of demographics, resources and life stress, Bonanno, Galea, Bucciarelli and Vlahov (2007) suggest that no single factor is responsible for resilience. Rather, there is a 'coalescence' of various aspects.

Certain factors, like personality, may be relatively stable over time, whilst others will vary (Hobfoll, 2002).

## Personality

Although there is a widespread assumption that personality is responsible for resilience, Bonanno et al. (2011) warn against overestimating its role. Nevertheless, as Bonanno et al. (2011) discuss, in studies that have measured personality both pre- and post-PTE, high scores on perceived control (Ullman & Newcombe, 1999) and resilience trait (Ong, Fulluer-Rowell & Bonanno, 2010) or low scores on negative affectivity (Weems et al., 2010) and ruminative response style (Nolen-Hoeksema & Morrow, 1991) have been associated with enhanced post-event outcomes. Ego strength and optimism (Farber, Schwartz, Schaper, Moonen & McDaniel, 2000) have also been associated with resilience. However, caution must be employed because, as Tennen and Affleck (1999) point out, in studies where personality is measured post-event, apparent personality characteristics may in fact be an outcome of coping with adversity.

## Environmental factors

Personality combines with aspects of the individual's environment in facilitating resilience. Of the numerous factors involved, those of social and economic resources have to date received the greatest attention (e.g., Hobfoll, 2002). People who cope well with trauma have often been embedded in a supportive social context (Lepore & Revenson, 2006). This support can take many forms, ranging from emotional to informational, as described by Kaniasty and Norris (2009). Greater social capital, with greater access to social support, leads, in the majority of cases, to resilience in adversity (Saegert, Thompson & Warren, 2001).

Access to economic resources is often associated with resilience, with increased availability correlated with better adjustment (Brewin, Andrews & Valentine, 2000). Unfortunately, it is often the case that PTEs result in a decreased availability of resources (Hobfoll, 2002), which in turn reduces the prevalence of resilience in the affected population (Bonanno et al., 2007). Furthermore, war often occurs during or as a result of a breakdown in civil order, so many of those experiencing it may have previously been subjected to hardship, followed by limited support after the traumatic event.

## Previous stressors

There is mixed information regarding previous experience of life stress and its association with resilience (Bonanno et al., 2011). For example, research has linked past and current stress with increased risk of PTSD (Brewin et al.,

2000) and attendant decreased likelihood of resilience (Bonanno et al., 2007). However, Bonanno, Brewin, Kaniasty and LaGreca (2010) and Silverman and LaGreca (2002) have noted that in the case of disasters, prior experience confers a better outcome.

### Agency and self-efficacy

Agency and self-efficacy factors have often been associated with resilience (Luthar, 2006). Positive self-esteem protected children (aged 9–13 years) against PTSD following the 9/11 attacks in New York (Lengua, Long, Smith & Meltzoff, 2005). In their study of child soldiers, Betancourt et al. (2010) found that those who had survived rape during captivity had greater confidence than other child soldiers, possibly a reflection of having managed to endure such hardships.

### A priori beliefs and worldviews

Children who grow up in a loving and responsive environment are more likely to develop a positive self-image and positive expectations of the future. Such individuals are more likely to be resilient to adversity (Ahmann, 2002; Masten & Coatsworth, 1998).

### Faith and spirituality

Whilst established as influential in resilience in general, spirituality holds particular saliency in the context of war and conflict (Crawford, Wright & Masten, 2006). According to Klasen et al. (2010), former child soldiers who demonstrated post-traumatic resilience also declared a greater perceived spiritual support. This may reflect the significance of belief systems in providing coherence and meaning to life in devastating circumstances (Palmeiri, Danetti-Nisim, Galea, Johnson & Hobfoll, 2008; Wright, Masten & Narayan, 2012).

### Acculturation skills

For those who move to new cultures as a result of conflict, greater acculturation and language skills are associated with better adaptation and apparent resilience (Wright et al., 2012).

### The physical environment

Research on ill health and bereavement has shown that in such adversity, environmental design can promote well-being (Stokols, 1992). Whether this can be extrapolated to promoting resilience is yet to be explored.

## Types of resilience

Lepore and Revenson (2006) expand the idea of resilience to trauma by suggesting that the term is often used to capture different concepts. This, they maintain, reflects the complex nature of the construct:

(a) *Recovery*

> Lepore and Revenson (2006) take a stance somewhat contrary to Bonanno's (2004) suggestion that for individuals to be described as resilient they must demonstrate either an almost immediate recovery or a complete absence of any negative reactions. Instead, Lepore and Revenson (2006) propose that even those who are slow to resume normal functioning can be described as resilient compared to those who never recover at all.

(b) *Resistance*

> Here, Lepore and Revenson (2006) are in line with Bonanno (2004), describing resilience as including those who exhibit normal functioning before, during and after a stressor. However, this form of resilience does not sit well with prevailing psychological or cultural expectations. There has, therefore, been a tendency to pathologize this type of response, despite evidence to the contrary (Wortman & Silver, 1989). Such mistakenness has resulted in the overprescription of unnecessary and inappropriate interventions in resistant individuals.

(c) *Reconfiguration*

> Individuals exhibit this type of resilience when they are able to reconfigure their cognitions, beliefs and behaviours in a way that enables them to adapt to traumatic experiences and possibly withstand future traumas (Lepore & Revenson, 2006). Reconfiguration is similar to post-traumatic growth (PTG). However, whereas PTG refers to positive changes, reconfiguration can include both negative and positive changes.

Resilience is a widespread human response to trauma. It is a dynamic process, leading to adaptive outcomes in the face of adversity (Lepore & Revenson, 2006). Resilience is not simply a personality trait, rather it is a multidimensional concept: a product of the individual, his or her life experiences and current life context. Due to its dynamic properties, individuals may experience resilience in some situations but not others. It should be noted that it is often found that the greater the trauma, the greater the resources and will of survivors to continue with their lives (Erbes, 2004).

Whilst resilience is the most prevalent response to trauma, post-traumatic stress disorder (PTSD) has received greater focus in the literature. This is due in part to the initial misconception of resilience as an unusual rather than a common response. More importantly, the potentially destructive nature of PTSD required it to be examined and addressed.

## Post-traumatic stress disorder (PTSD)

As far back as the ancient writing of Homer's *Iliad*, the psychological con-sequences of trauma have been well documented. Despite this, the study of traumatic response is a relatively recent discipline. In the military field, it was long recognized that well-adjusted individuals could develop acute stress symp-toms following harrowing events (Shepherd, 2001). Descriptive terms devel-oped included 'shell shock', 'war neurosis' and 'combat fatigue'. It was initially believed that symptoms would dissipate when the individual was removed from conflict (Wilson, 1994). However, studies with veterans of twentieth-century wars, particularly those of the Vietnam War, proved otherwise; that such distress could be a long-lasting disorder. Subsequent work into the impact of other life stressors, such as rape (Burgess & Holmstrom, 1974), together with information from Vietnam veterans, World War II veterans and concentration camp survi-vors produced the diagnosis of PTSD. This concept of PTSD has done much to assist in the recognition of the needs of survivors, who were previously misun-derstood, stigmatized or ignored. In 1980, the American Psychiatric Association (APA) added PTSD to the third edition of its *Diagnostic and Statistical Manual of Mental Disorders* (*DSM-III*). The most recent version, *DSM-V*, has an extensive description of diagnostic criteria for PTSD, which can be summarized as follows (based on American Psychiatric Association, 2013, pp. 271–72):

1   Exposure to actual or threatened death, serious injury or sexual violence.
2   Presence of one (or more) of the following intrusion symptoms associated with the traumatic event(s), beginning after the traumatic event(s) occurred: spontaneous memories of the traumatic event, recurrent dreams related to it, flashbacks, other intense or prolonged psychological distress, or marked physiological reactions to trauma-related stimuli.
3   Persistent avoidance of stimuli associated with the traumatic event(s), begin-ning after the traumatic event(s) occurred, as evidenced by one of the fol-lowing: avoidance of distressing memories, thoughts, feelings or external reminders of the event.
4   Negative alterations in cognitions and mood associated with the traumatic event(s), beginning or worsening after the traumatic event(s) occurred, as evidenced by two (or more) of the following: persistent negative beliefs about the self or the world, a persistent and distorted sense of blame of self or others, persistent negative trauma-related emotions, constricted affect, estrangement from others, a markedly diminished interest in activities or the inability to remember key aspects of the event.
5   Marked alterations in arousal and reactivity associated with the traumatic event(s), beginning or worsening after the traumatic event(s) occurred, as evidenced by two (or more) of the following: aggressive behaviour, reckless or self-destructive behaviour, sleep disturbances, hyper-vigilance, exagger-ated startle response or concentration problems.

6    Duration of the disturbance is more than one month.
7    The disturbance causes clinically significant distress or impairment in social, occupational or other areas of functioning.
8    The disturbance is not attributable to the physiological effects of a substance (e.g., medication, alcohol) or another medical condition.

In addition to psychological symptoms, there are considerable interpersonal and social consequences. These include an increased divorce rate, difficulties in parenting (which may have greater impact on the child than the war trauma itself) (Dias, Sales, Cardoso & Kleber, 2014; Lambert, Holzer & Hasbun, 2014; Olema, Catani, Ertl, Saile & Neuner, 2014), physical health problems and decreased earning potential (Jordan et al., 1992; Schnurr & Green, 2004; Walker et al., 2003). Cascading socio-emotional and even genetic effects can be observed in subsequent generations of PTSD sufferers (Masten & Narayan, 2012). This highlights the significance of PTSD both to the individual and to society at large.

## Prevalence

As mentioned in our discussion of resilience, even though exposure to potentially traumatic events (PTE) is quite common, development of PTSD is rare, with rates varying between populations, as examined by Johnson and Thompson (2008) and Keane, Marshall and Taft (2006).

### The general population

In studies in the United States, Kessler, Berglund, Demler, Jin and Walters (2005) found an overall lifetime PTSD prevalence of 6.8 per cent, making it the fifth most common psychiatric condition in the country. In an earlier study where overall prevalence was found to be 7.8 per cent, gender differences were observed, with women (10.4 per cent) more than twice as likely as men (5.0 per cent) to develop PTSD over their lifetime (Kessler, Sonnega, Bromet, Hughes & Nelson, 1995). Similar rates and gender splits have been observed in many populations.

### Combatants

Military personnel are, unsurprisingly, at high risk of developing PTSD due to their increased exposure to conflict-associated trauma. A major study of Vietnam veterans and civilian comparators showed that 64 per cent of Vietnam veterans were exposed to traumatic events compared to 45 per cent of civilians (Kulka et al., 1990). Unlike many populations, here the gender split was different, with 15 per cent of men and 9 per cent of women meeting PTSD criteria. It is likely that this gender difference reflects the roles women held in the military at the time. In more recent wars, for example the Gulf Wars, PTSD was observed in 4 per cent of men and 9 per cent of women (Wolfe, Brown & Kelley, 1993).

## Refugees

As discussed by Johnson and Thompson (2008), high rates of PTSD have been found amongst refugees affected by war trauma. These range from 23.5 per cent (Eytan, Gex-Fabry, Toscani, Deroo & Bovier, 2004) to 65 per cent (Ai, Peterson & Ubelhor, 2002). Turner, Bowie, Dunn, Shapo and Yule (2003) argue that this variation is due to methodology, with self-report measures overestimating prevalence whilst interview techniques indicate lower rates. It must also be remembered that at the point of investigation, many refugees are in the midst of the asylum process and it may assist their case to exaggerate symptoms. Nonetheless, rates are higher than in the general population. This could be due to the extended duration of trauma and the lack of socio-emotional support available to refugees (Mazur, Chahraoui & Bissler, 2014).

### Theories of PTSD

According to Brewin & Holmes (2003), early theories fell into three categories:

- **Social cognitive theories** focus on the way trauma breaches existing mental structures and on innate mechanisms for reconciling incompatible information with previous beliefs, e.g., Stress Response Theory (Horowitz, 1976).
- **Conditioning theories** concern learnt associations and avoidance behaviour, e.g., Keane and Barlow (2002).
- **Information processing theories** centre on the encoding, storage and recall of fear-inducing events and their associated stimuli and responses, e.g., Litz and Keane (1989).

These initial theories provided useful insights into PTSD. However, they were restricted by the small amount of data available at the time.

More recently, as Brewin and Holmes (2003) discuss, theories have been developed with a broader scope:

- **Emotional processing theory** elaborates the relationship between PTSD and knowledge available prior to, during and after the trauma. Those with more rigid views would be more vulnerable to PTSD (e.g., Foa & Rothbaum, 1998). Such views could reinforce critical negative schemata involving incompetence and danger underlying PTSD.
- **Dual representation theory** states that pathological responses (e.g., vivid re-experiencing) arise when trauma memories become dissociated from the ordinary memory system, so that two memory systems operate in parallel, with one taking precedence over the other at different times. Recovery involves the transforming of these dissociated memories into ordinary, narrative memories (e.g., van der Kolk & van der Hart, 1991).

- **The cognitive model** draws attention to the PTSD paradox that individuals feel anxious about the future even though the trauma is situated in the past. Ehlers and Clark (2000) proposed that pathological responses to trauma arise when individuals process the traumatic information in a way that produces a sense of current threat. They suggest that there are two principal mechanisms causing this effect – negative appraisal of the trauma, and the nature of the trauma memory itself. Negative appraisal can become increasingly likely according to the thought processes (e.g., 'mental defeat') occurring during the trauma.

Criticism of these theories includes their reliance on the Western concept of 'self' (Bracken, 1998). It is widely acknowledged that many non-Western cultures devise a sense of self through their societal roles, and therefore Western ideas of PTSD may be less relevant. As trauma not only impacts a person's beliefs but also affects their social world (Brewin & Holmes, 2003), theories may need to be expanded to embrace this aspect more readily.

### Risk factors of PTSD

Despite many people experiencing trauma, the majority will not develop PTSD. The inherent complexity of the disorder means that a single, definitive reason as to why certain individuals develop PTSD cannot be determined. Numerous studies have identified various risk factors that enhance the chances of PTSD. Such is the heterogeneity and reality of life that these factors are most likely to interact in varying degrees to produce a cumulative effect. These are described below, as reviewed by Johnson and Thompson (2008) and Keane, Marshall and Taft (2006).

#### Preexisting factors

It is important to recognize that a predisposition to exposure to traumatic events and a predisposition to developing PTSD are separate entities that are difficult to separate in research methodologies.

Familial psychopathology. Despite early animal work suggesting a genetic component in sensitivity to environmental stress (Anisman, Grimmer, Irwin, Remington & Sklar, 1979), there is little evidence of a genetic influence on the development of PTSD following combat trauma (Roy-Byrne et al., 2004), although Stein, Jang, Taylor, Vernon and Lively (2002) suggested that such an association exists in the case of noncombatants experiencing interpersonal violence. A family history of psychopathology predicts a small increase in PTSD, the effect being greater for noncombatants than combatants. Nevertheless, it would appear that, overall, environmental factors have a greater influence than genetic influences.

Demographic factors. It should be noted that these factors may serve as proxies for other issues, such as social burden and life adversity.

Sex: Although historically men have appeared to be exposed to more trauma, women have had a higher prevalence of PTSD. This may reflect the type of trauma women are more likely to be exposed to (such as sexual assault). However, controlling for this, Breslau, Chilcoat, Kessler, Peterson and Lucia (1999) still found that women are more at risk of developing PTSD than men. Johnson and Thompson (2008) reviewed studies of gender differences in civilian response to war and discovered that in the majority, women were more likely to develop PTSD than men. This was later supported in a meta-analysis by Furr, Comer, Edmunds and Kendall (2010).

Age: No effect of age has been seen amongst women. However, a strong positive correlation has been observed in men, possibly due to the increased exposure to trauma over the life span (Kessler, 1995). In combat zones, male civilians over the age of 65 have been found to be at an increased risk of developing PTSD (Cardozo, Vergara, Agani & Gotway, 2000).

Psychopathology prior to the trauma. The prior existence of a psychiatric condition has been identified as a risk factor for PTSD in several studies (e.g., Ozer, Best, Lipsey & Weiss, 2003). Depression particularly has a significant effect. In addition, one must remember that the presence of psychopathology may also lead to increased exposure to trauma.

### Factors relating to the traumatic event itself

Unsurprisingly, the nature of the event will have an effect on PTSD development. Most theories suggest a dose response between symptom and trauma severity. In addition, several variables occurring during the trauma are also important, such as cognitions during the trauma, physiology, and affect.

Trauma severity (dose-response relationship). As mentioned above, studies (including cross-cultural) have found associations between the severity of a traumatic event and PTSD symptom severity. A particular example of increased severity is that those inflicted with physical injuries are at greater risk of more severe PTSD.

Perceived life threat and peritraumatic emotional response. A small association was observed by Ozer et al. (2003) between perceived life threat and PTSD, which increased with time elapsed since trauma. The relationship between peritraumatic emotional responses (e.g., helplessness, fear, etc.) can explain up to 67 per cent of PTSD symptoms six months later (Tucker, Pfefferbaum, Nixon & Dickson, 2000). Of particular impact were negative appraisal of trauma, low self-efficacy and an external locus of control. Individual differences in peritraumatic emotional responses may also be due to differences in meaning assigned to the traumatic event.

Peritraumatic dissociation. Dissociation includes symptoms such as an altered sense of time and 'blanking out'. Peritraumatic dissociation was found by

Schnurr and Green (2004) to play a role in maintaining PTSD. Gershuny, Cloitre and Otto (2003) go on to suggest that peritraumatic dissociation may be part of the panic process, with the cognitive elements of panicking potentially overriding the dissociative elements in their relative importance to PTSD development. In general, cognitive variables such as cognitive processing during the trauma, trauma memory disorganization, persistent dissociation and negative interpretations of trauma memories each predicted PTSD symptoms beyond objective and subjective measures of stressor severity (Keane et al., 2006).

### Post-trauma factors

Social support. Social support has received the most attention in this arena. In several studies, increased social support was related to decreased PTSD severity, an effect which increased with the amount of time which had elapsed since the trauma (Ozer et al., 2003). This effect was particularly visible in war combatants.

### Controversy

The validity of PTSD diagnoses was called into question in the 1970s and 1980s (Goodwin & Guze, 1984). Whilst much of this debate has since dissipated, controversy remains. It is currently centred upon the definition of trauma, whether PTSD should be defined by symptoms alone, and whether it is in fact a product of social construction and is instead a normal response which dissipates over time. There is also debate concerning distortion in trauma recollection, the recovery of memories of childhood sexual abuse, and the reliability of PTSD theoretical models (McNally, 2003).

In summary, although it affects only a minority, PTSD is the most common psychopathological response to trauma. Higher rates are observed amongst women than men and appear greater in lesser-developed countries. This may be due to differences in social structures or to the availability of resources following large-scale traumatic events. It may also be explained by issues concerning research methodology, particularly in overgeneralizing concepts across cultures. Individual factors appear influential in determining who develops PTSD. Demographic factors appear to correlate with PTSD but many may act as proxies of other variables, such as access to resources and life adversity. In fact, life adversity confers a high degree of risk for PTSD. The most significant risks of all appear to be the characteristics of the trauma involved, the peritraumatic response of the individual, and the availability of post-trauma social support. As will be examined in later chapters, religious and cultural beliefs have a protective influence over PTSD, as does a sense of preparedness for the forthcoming trauma (Meichenbaum, 1994), although this is rarely available. A danger of the PTSD diagnosis is that it may constrain recovery and dominate the personal narrative. A diagnosis may indeed severely constrain elaboration of the construct system and, thereby, recovery (see section on personal construct psychology and its approach to trauma, below).

## Post-traumatic growth (PTG)

Like PTSD, post-traumatic growth (PTG) has been well documented through the ages. Throughout history, many philosophies have recognized that personal gain can be found through suffering (Tedeschi & Calhoun, 1995). Indeed, such ideas are central to many contemporary religions. The study of PTG as a specific issue is very recent but it is now well established that traumatic events can promote personal growth and positive change (Joseph & Linley, 2006).

Post-traumatic growth has been defined by Tedeschi and Calhoun (1995) as the 'positive change experienced as a result of the struggle with trauma', and represents a response that goes beyond a person's previous level of functioning (Joseph & Linley, 2006). Three general domains where growth can occur have been identified (Tedeschi & Calhoun, 2006):

*Changed perception of self: strength and new possibilities*

- personal strength in the face of vulnerability
- embarking on new life paths or interests as a result of traumatic experience

*Relating to others*

- greater connection and intimacy with other people
- increased compassion for others' suffering
- increased freedom to be oneself

*Changed philosophy of life: priorities, appreciation and spirituality*

- change in priorities
- appreciation of 'the small things' in life
- existential and spiritual changes providing a greater sense of purpose and understanding.

Post-traumatic growth is far from a universal experience. Estimates of PTG prevalence are somewhat varied. Most commonly reported rates range from sizeable minorities (30–40%) to majorities (60–80%) (Linley & Joseph, 2004), although different measuring techniques have been used to measure a concept that is notoriously difficult to quantify (Tedeschi & Calhoun, 2006). Caution must be exercised when discussing high rates of prevalence, due to the potentially negative impact on individuals who do not experience such growth during their struggle with trauma.

### Theories of post-traumatic growth

According to Splevins, Cohen, Bowley and Joseph (2010), there are two major theories of post-traumatic growth – the **Functional Descriptive Model** of

Tedeschi and Calhoun (1996), and Joseph and Linley's (2006) **Organismic Valuing Process Theory**. Like the dominant theories of PTSD, these have been developed within the concepts of the Western world. Also aligned to the PTSD theories is their suggestion that adversity challenges an individual's assumptions about the world. This conflict between the pre- and post-trauma worldviews causes psychological distress (Splevins et al., 2010). PTG theories propose that an individual's ability to integrate such new information into existing belief systems allows a propensity for growth. Indeed, recent work by Shakespeare-Finch and Lurie-Beck (2014) has described a relationship between PTG and PTSD symptoms, suggesting that both positive and negative post-trauma outcomes can co-occur. (A focus only on PTSD symptoms may limit or slow recovery and mask the potential for growth.)

### Factors involved in post-traumatic growth

Correlations have been established between post-traumatic growth and various psychological, social, environmental and demographic variables (Meyerson, Grant, Smith Carter & Kilmer, 2011). Positive correlates include optimism, social support and spirituality (Prati & Pietrantoni, 2009). Other factors influencing PTG are the individual's subjective experience of the event, education level and personality (extraversion, openness to experience, agreeableness, conscientiousness, self-efficacy, hardiness, optimism and high self-esteem are associated with growth) (Linley and Joseph, 2004). Evidence demonstrates that (older) women, individuals from ethnic minorities and younger adults experience most post-traumatic growth. There is some evidence to suggest that the longer the time since the traumatic event, the greater the extent of PTG (Cordova, Cunningham, Carlson & Andrykowski, 2001). However, it is unlikely that it is the actual amount of time passed that influences PTG; rather, it is the intervening events and processes.

There is now much evidence demonstrating that many individuals can experience growth following a traumatic event and that this growth can be mediated by various factors.

## The significance of cultural context in trauma

The importance of cultural context in the diagnosis of PTSD is emphasized by the American Psychiatric Association (2013) in the *DSM-V*. People's fundamental assumptions, their ability to modify these post-trauma, and the type of social support they receive are all shaped by local culture (McMillen, 2004). Bracken (1998) stresses the importance of contextual factors in determining responses to trauma. These factors should not be considered secondary – rather, they are fundamental, as local realities (social, political and cultural) combine to establish the meaning of an event and the individual response. Reactions to trauma may have different values or meanings in different cultures. A response may be inaccurately diagnosed as distressing when presenting in a different setting to where it was first described.

Spirituality is an area of particular relevance in Sierra Leone, where many people have a strong belief in God (Muslim 60%, Christianity 20%, animism 20%). The belief that God will take care of them or that God's will takes precedence gives meaning to their world. It assists in their resilience to the many traumatic events the country has tragically suffered and continues to endure.

Despite the majority of contemporary wars being located in non-Western countries, Western ideas of trauma currently dominate. The world as it appears to both will be different, and one must not be privileged over the other. Caution must be taken with PTSD, for example, which may be thought of as reflecting a Western medicalization of trauma response. Such a model may have only limited relevance to non-Western populations. Contextual considerations are particularly important in the case of international refugees. In addition to the actual trauma, numerous other factors interact, including the disruption of social structure, emotional support and financial resources.

## Personal construct psychology and its approach to trauma

Human progress through life is guided by the ability to anticipate and predict experiences. Personal construct psychology (PCP) (Kelly, 1955) suggests that this is done by people acting like scientists, constantly devising, testing and revising personal hypotheses to help make sense of the changing world and anticipate future experiences. These hypotheses are derived from our personal constructs, the ways in which we discriminate between and give meaning to events. Personal constructs may be highly idiosyncratic or widely shared, and they vary in their importance to the construing of one's life, with some (core constructs) being central to one's identity (Winter, 1992). All constructs are 'bipolar', as Kelly (1955) argued that, for example, 'good' only has meaning when related to 'bad', but the particular choices of contrasts between poles are unique to the individual. For example, one person's construct of 'good/bad' may be to another 'good/mean'. Constructs are organized into a hierarchical system, again unique to the individual, with superordinate constructs subsuming subordinate. Consequently, although individuals may draw upon commonly or culturally shared ideas, they will ultimately develop construct systems that are idiosyncratic, and they will consequently experience, and respond to, similar situations in different ways.

The predictions derived from our construct systems may be validated or invalidated by subsequent events, and this and any resulting changes in construing will be accompanied with the experience of emotion. For example, if individuals find that their constructs do not enable them to make sense of events, they will experience anxiety. If they become aware that core aspects of their construct system are likely to change comprehensively and imminently, they will feel threatened. If they find themselves behaving in a way which is very different from how they have always seen their role in relation to others, they will experience guilt. Individuals may employ various strategies to deal with invalidation. For example, construing may be 'loosened' so that predictions become vaguer and therefore less vulnerable to invalidation. Conversely, it may be 'tightened', with predictions becoming more precise. Individuals may 'constrict' their world to those events that they can predict; or, conversely, 'dilate' it in an attempt to develop a way of construing the new experiences. Alternatively, the approach adopted may be one of 'hostility', which Kelly (1955) viewed in terms of the person extorting evidence for invalidated predictions rather than reconstruing in response to invalidation. For Kelly (1955), psychological disorders are characterized by the person repeatedly using a particular construction despite consistent invalidation. They may also be viewed in terms of an imbalanced use of the strategies described above: for example, persistent tightening, loosening, constriction, or dilation (Winter, 2003).

Experiences that are described as traumatic, like warfare for most people, are those that shatter long-held expectations and result in the individual struggling to make sense of what the event means about the self and the world in general. Such events cannot be understood in terms of the individual's preexisting construct system; rather, they violate or disrupt core beliefs and assumptions. Personal construct psychology emphasizes that the individual's reaction needs to be understood, not in terms of the traumatic event itself, but in the context of their personal construct system.

Sewell et al. (1996), on the basis of research with war veterans, proposed that PTSD is more than a disruption of an individual's assumptions about the world and the self. Rather, they suggested, it also involves structural changes in the construct system. They advanced the idea that trauma produces isolated construct classes that cannot integrate into the rest of the construct system. They suggest that this manifests in two ways. First, the constructs affecting the memory of the traumatic event are impaired, so that traumatized individuals cannot integrate the sensations and thoughts that occurred during the trauma. Combat victims are thus often unable to put together a 'good story' of what happened. Second, the traumatic event is not incorporated within superordinate constructs. It is not absorbed into the system hierarchy and subsequently construed in comparison to other negative life events. As we have seen, experiences like this, for which the individual has no relevant constructs available, create anxiety (Kelly 1955), part of the PTSD syndrome. Sewell et al. (1996) hypothesized, to encompass other symptomatology of PTSD (such as depression, social avoidance, intrusive thoughts), that a dissociated construct or construct subsystem has developed in response to the traumatic event. Such isolated constructs/construct subsystems are unstable and have a propensity for what Kelly (1955) termed 'slot movement' (Space & Cromwell, 1980). This refers to the movement from one pole of a construct to the other for a particular element, such as 'self'. This could be from a positive to negative meaning, or vice versa. This instability enables the individual to incorporate new information without developing new constructs. It is thought to be responsible for mood disturbance, as observed in PTSD. Sewell et al. (1996) also propose that there is an interactive relationship between the trauma that is construed in the isolated construct subsystem and trauma experiences for which constructs are never developed. As mentioned earlier, the latter would result in anxiety, and this anxiety might then initiate slot movement within the isolated trauma-related subsystem. The resulting mood disturbance could subsequently produce further anxiety due to an inability to construe the mood shift. This cyclical outcome could ultimately lead to a catastrophic or panic response.

Findings consistent with this model of PTSD were also obtained from a study of witnesses of a mass murder (Sewell et al., 1996), and the model has been further elaborated by Sewell (1997) and Sewell and Williams (2000). They detailed at least three possible responses to trauma: *constructive bankruptcy* – in which there are no dimensions of meaning available to place the trauma in context; *dissociated construction* – one or more constructions are created that are primitively used to construe the trauma but which do not relate well to the rest of the individual's construct system; *elaborative growth* – only minor adjustments are made to the construct system, the traumatic experience is rapidly accommodated and there is no 'traumatization'. When constructive bankruptcy or dissociated construction ensue, then post-traumatic stress disorder is more likely to be seen. Sewell and Williams (2000) suggest that recovery from PTSD occurs when constructs are developed that can be integrated into the individual's meaning ('construct') system. Sewell and Williams (2000) also considered which domains of construal are affected by trauma. At least two domains are affected, events and persons (social world). *Event disruption* occurs when a trauma invalidates expectations of how the world should be. This is a central aspect in many presentations of post-traumatic stress. War and conflict invalidate, particularly for civilians, expectations that the world is safe, life is fair and human bodies remain intact. *Social disruption* involves the invalidation of anticipations regarding 'how and with whom am I socially related'. Social disruption is often observed as a secondary event to a difficulty in construing or processing an event. However, in post-traumatic reactions, it can be a primary occurrence. In the majority of cases, there are problems in both the event and social domains, although one is likely to predominate in clinical presentation.

Sermpezis and Winter (2009) have challenged the model of PTSD proposed by Sewell et al. (1996), suggesting that the results on which this was based, indicating a lack of integration of the trauma into the construct system, were a methodological artifact. Their findings suggest the opposite conclusion to Sewell et al., namely that traumatic events appear to be more integrated than non-traumatic, that they have stronger connections with associated constructs and that they occupy superordinate positions within the individual's personal construct system. This supports the conceptualization of trauma as a reference point within a person's autobiographical knowledge base, which has implications for the rest of the construct system and their self-narrative.

In experiencing trauma, one's sense of self can be disturbed. As indicated in personal construct studies of survivors of childhood sexual abuse (e.g., Harter, Alexander & Neimeyer, 1988), the self can come to be seen as very different from other people. From a constructivist viewpoint, the sense of self can be seen as a narrative achievement (Neimeyer & Levitt, 2001). People construe meaning in their life experiences by punctuating the seamless flow of events and organizing them according to recurrent themes (Kelly, 1995). This in turn provides a scaffold for the 'plot' of one's life story (Neimeyer, 2000). The self-narrative thereby provides a means of assimilating experience into the individual's construct system. When traumatic events challenge their adequacy, constructs must undergo revision to accommodate the changed circumstances (Neimeyer, 2005). The trauma may be radically incoherent to the plot of the individual's prior life narrative and may also invalidate core emotional themes. It may create a 'traumatic self' around which the self-narrative subsequently develops, integrating subsequent life experiences that are emotionally congruent with it. That is, it can become a dominant narrative which 'colonizes' the sense of self, reducing the options of identity to those that are problem-saturated (White & Epston, 1990). This dominance can culminate in a post-traumatic identity which is consolidated at personal and social levels, acting as an interpretive framework for integrating subsequent life experiences and relating and enacting them with others (Neimeyer, Herrero & Botella, 2006). A person who is unable to integrate the trauma into their construct system may dissociate the traumatic memory, excluding aspects from both conscious awareness and the narration of their experience in a social context. The result is a silent story that resists integration into the self-narrative (Neimeyer, 2000). Holding the memory in this form, unassimilated into the construct system, can serve defensive functions at the personal level (Stiles, Osatuke, Glick & Mackay, 2004) in addition to protection from potential social exclusion. Conversely, the individual may develop an inability to forget the most distressing and intrusive memories, causing great distress.

## Conclusions

Despite its recent establishment as a specific discipline, we are rapidly gaining knowledge of the sequelae of war trauma. Whilst resilience is the most common response, post-traumatic stress disorder (PTSD) remains a painful outcome. The type of post-traumatic response experienced by a person is determined by individual, societal and environmental factors. With the increasing and changing nature of conflict around the world, knowledge of its psychological impact, both negative and positive, is required to fully support those who have survived such terrible atrocities.

# References

Ahmann, E. (2002) Promoting positive parenting: An annotated bibliography. *Pediatric Nursing,* 28(4): 382–385.

Ai, A. L., Peterson, C., Ubelhor, D. (2002) War-related trauma and symptoms of posttraumatic stress disorder among adult Kosovar refugees. *Journal of Traumatic Stress,* 15: 157–160.

American Psychiatric Association (2013) *Diagnostic and statistical manual of mental disorders* (5th ed.). Washington, DC: APA.

Anisman, H., Grimmer, L., Irwin, J., Remington, G., Sklar, L. S. (1979) Escape performance after inescapable shock and selectively bred lines of mice: Response maintenance and catecholamine activity. *Journal of Comparative and Physiological Psychology,* 93: 229–241.

Betancourt, T. S., Borisova, I. I., Williams, T. P., Brennan, R. T., Whitfield, T. H., De La Soudiere, M., Williamson, J., Gilman, S. E. (2010) Sierra Leone's former child soldiers: A follow-up study of psychosocial adjustment and community reintegration. *Child Development,* 81: 1077–1095.

Bonanno, G. A. (2004) Loss, trauma and human resilience: Have we underestimated the human capacity to thrive after extremely adverse events? *American Psychologist,* 59: 20–28.

Bonanno, G. A. (2012) Uses and abuses of the resilience construct: Loss, trauma and health-related adversities. *Science & Medicine,* 74: 753–756.

Bonanno, G. A., Brewin, C. R., Kaniasty, K., LaGreca, A.M. (2010) Weighing the cost of disaster: Consequences, risks and resilience in individuals, families and communities. *Psychological Science in the Public Interest,* 11(1): 1–49.

Bonanno, G. A., Galea, S., Bucciarelli, A., Vlahov, D. (2007) What predicts psychological resilience after disaster? The role of demographics, resources and life stress. *Journal of Consulting and Clinical Psychology,* 75: 671–682.

Bonanno, G. A., Westphal, M., Mancini, A. D. (2011) Resilience to loss and potential trauma. *Annual Review of Clinical Psychology,* 7: 511–535.

Bracken, P. J. (1998) Hidden agendas: Deconstructing posttraumatic stress disorder. In P. J. Bracken, C. Petty (Eds.), *Rethinking the trauma of war* (pp. 38–59). London/New York: Free Association Books.

Breslau, N., Chilcoat, H. D., Kessler, R. C., Peterson, E. L., Lucia, V. C. (1999) Vulnerability to assaultive violence: Further specification of the sex difference in post-traumatic stress disorder. *Psychological Medicine,* 298: 813–821.

Brewin, C. R., Andrews, B., Valentine, J. D. (2000) Meta-analysis of risk factors for posttraumatic stress disorder in trauma-exposed adults. *Journal of Consulting and Clinical Psychology,* 68: 748–766.

Brewin, C. R., Holmes, E. A. (2003) Psychological theories of posttraumatic stress disorder. *Clinical Psychology Review,* 23: 339–376.

Burgess, A. W., Holmstrom, L. (1974) Rape trauma syndrome. *American Journal of Psychiatry,* 131: 981–986.

Cardozo, B. L., Vergara, A., Agani, F., Gotway, C. A. (2000) Mental health, social functioning and attitudes of Kosovar Albanians following the war in Kosovo. *The Journal of the American Medical Association,* 284: 569–577.

Cordova, M. J., Cunningham, L.L.C., Carlson, C. R., Andrykowski, M. (2001) Posttraumatic growth following breast cancer: A controlled comparison study. *Health Psychology,* 20: 176–185.

Crawford, E., Wright, M. O., Masten, A. S. (2006) Resilience and spirituality in youth. In E. C. Roehlkepartain, P. E. King, L. Wagener, P. L. Benson (Eds.), *The handbook of spiritual development in childhood and adolescence* (pp. 355–370). Thousand Oaks, CA: Sage.

Dias, A., Sales, L., Cardoso, R. M., Kleber, R. (2014) Childhood maltreatment in adult off-spring of Portuguese war veterans with and without PTSD. *European Journal of Psychotraumatology,* 5: 20198.

Ehlers, A., Clark, D. M. (2000) A cognitive model of posttraumatic stress disorder. *Behaviour Research and Therapy,* 38: 319–345.

Erbes, C. (2004) Our constructions of trauma: A dialectical perspective. *Journal of Constructivist Psychology,* 17: 201–220.

Eytan, A., Gex-Fabry, M., Toscani, L., Deroo, L., Bovier, P. A. (2004) Determinants of postconflict symptoms in Albanian Kosovans. *Journal of Nervous and Mental Disease,* 192: 257–262.

Farber, P., Schwartz, J. A., Schaper, P. E., Moonen, D. J., McDaniel, J. S. (2000) Resilience factors associated with adaptation to HIV disease. *Psychosomatics,* 41 (2): 140–146.

Foa, E. B., Rothbaum, B. O. (1998) *Treating the trauma of rape: Cognitive behavioural therapy for PTSD.* New York: Guilford Press.

Furr, J. M., Comer, J. S., Edmunds, J. M., Kendall, P. C. (2010) Disasters and youth: A meta-analytic examination of posttraumatic stress. *Journal of Consulting and Clinical Psychology,* 78(6): 765–780.

Gershuny, B .S., Cloitre, M., Otto, M. W. (2003) Peritraumatic dissociation and PTSD severity: Do event-related fears about death and control mediate their relation? *Behavioural Research and Therapy,* 41: 157–166.

Goodwin, D. W., Guze, S. B. (1984) *Psychiatric diagnosis.* New York: Oxford University Press.

Harter, S. L., Alexander, P. C., Neimeyer, R. A. (1988) Long-term effects of incestuous child abuse in college women: Social adjustment, social cognition, and family characteristics. *Journal of Consulting and Clinical Psychology,* 56: 5–8.

Hobfoll, S. E. (2002) Social and psychological responses and adaptation. *Review of General Psychology,* 6: 307–324.

Hobfoll, S. E., Mancini, A. D., Hall, B. J., Canetti, D., Bonanno, G. A. (2011) The limits of resilience: Distress following chronic political violence among Palestinians. *Social Science & Medicine,* 72: 1400–1408.

Horowitz, M. J. (1976) *Stress response syndromes.* New York: Aronson.

Johnson, H., Thompson, A. (2008) The development and maintenance of post-traumatic stress disorder (PTSD) in civilian adult survivors of war trauma and torture: A review. *Clinical Psychology Review,* 28: 36–47.

Jordan, B. K., Marmar, C. R., Fairbank, J. A., Schlenger, W. E., Kulka, R. A., Hough, R. L., Weiss, D. S. (1992) Problems in families of male Vietnam veterans with posttraumatic stress disorder. *Journal of Consulting and Clinical Psychology,* 60: 916–926.

Joseph, S., Linley, P. A. (2006) Growth following adversity: Theoretical perspectives and implications for clinical practice. *Clinical Psychology Review,* 26: 1041–1053.

Kaniasty, K., Norris, G. H. (2009) Distinctions that matter: Received social support, perceived social support and social embeddedness after disasters. In Y. Neria, S. Galea, F. N. Norris (Eds.), *Mental health and disasters* (pp. 175–200). New York: Cambridge University Press.

Keane, M. K., Marshall, A. D., Taft, C. T. (2006) Posttraumatic stress disorder: Etiology, epidemiology and treatment outcome. *Annual Review of Clinical Psychology,* 2: 161–197.

Keane, T. M., Barlow, D. H. (2002) Posttraumatic stress disorder. In D. H. Barlow (Ed.), *Anxiety and its disorders* (2nd ed., pp. 418–453). New York: Guilford.

Kelly, G. A. (1955) *The psychology of personal constructs.* New York: Norton. (Reprinted by Routledge, 1991)

Kessler, R. C. (1995) The national comorbidity survey: Preliminary results and future directions. *International Journal of Methods in Psychiatric Research,* 5: 139–151.

Kessler, R. C., Berglund, P., Demler, O., Jin, R., Walters, E. E. (2005) Lifetime prevalence and age-of-onset distributions of DSM-IV disorders in the National Comorbidity Survey. *Archive of General Psychiatry,* 62: 592–602.

Kessler, R. C., Sonnega, A., Bromet, E., Hughes, M., Nelson, C. B. (1995) Posttraumatic stress disorder in the National Comorbidity Survey. *Archive of General Psychiatry,* 52: 1048–1060.

Klasen, F., Oettingen, G., Daniels, J., Post, M., Hoyer, C., Adam, H. (2010) Posttraumatic resilience in former Ugandan child soldiers. *Child Development,* 81(4): 1095–1112.

Kulka, R. A., Schlenger, W. E., Fairbank, J. A., Hough, R. L., Jordan, B. K. Marmar, Charles R., Weiss, Daniel S. (1990) *Trauma and the Vietnam war generation: Report of findings from the National Vietnam Veterans Readjustment Study.* New York: Brunner/Mazel.

Lambert, J. E., Holzer, J., Hasbun, A. (2014) Association between parents' PTSD severity and children's psychological distress: A meta-analysis. *Journal of Traumatic Stress,* 27(1): 9–17.

Lengua, L. J., Long, A. C., Smith, K. I., Meltzoff, A. N. (2005) Pre-attack symptomatology and temperament as predictors of children's responses to the September 11 terrorist attacks. *Journal of Child Psychology and Psychiatry,* 46(6): 631–645.

Lepore, S. J., Revenson, T. A. (2006) Resilience and posttraumatic growth: Recovery, resistance and reconfiguration. In L. G. Calhoun, R. G. Tedeschi (Eds.), *Handbook of posttraumatic growth: Research and practice* (pp. 24–46). Mahwah, NJ: Erlbaum.

Linley, P. A, Joseph, S. (2004) Positive change following adversity: A review. *Journal of Traumatic Stress,* 17: 11–21.

Litz, B. T., Keane, T. M. (1989) Information processing in anxiety disorders: Application to the understanding of posttraumatic stress disorder. *Clinical Psychology Review,* 9: 243–257.

Luthar, S. S. (2006) Resilience in development: A synthesis of research across five decades. In D. Cicchetti, D. J. Cohen (Eds.), *Developmental psychopathology. Vol. 3: Risk, disorder and adaptation* (pp. 739–795). Hoboken, NJ: Wiley.

Masten, A. S. (2001) Ordinary magic: resilience processes in development. *American Psychologist,* 56: 227–238.

Masten, A. S. (2011) Resilience in children threatened by extreme adversity: Frameworks for research, practice and translational symmetry. *Developmental Psychopathology,* 23(2): 141–145.

Masten, A. S., Coatsworth, J. D. (1998) The development of competence in favorable and unfavorable environments: Lessons from research on successful children. *American Psychologist,* 53(2): 205–220.

Masten, A. S., Narayan, A. J. (2012) Child development in the context of disaster, war and terrorism: Pathways of risk and resilience. *Annual Review of Psychology,* 63: 227–257.

Mazur, V. M., Chahraoui, K., Bissler, L. (2014) *Psychopathology of asylum seekers in Europe, trauma and defensive functioning.* Available at: http://europepmc.org/abstract/med/24661581 [Accessed 2 May 2015].

McMillen, J. (2004) Posttraumatic growth: What's it all about? *Psychology Inquiry,* 15: 48–52.

McNally, R. J. (2003) Progress and controversy in the study of posttraumatic stress disorder. *Annual Review of Psychology,* 54: 229–252.

Meichenbaum, D. (1994) *Clinical handbook/practical therapist manual for assessing and treating adults with post-traumatic stress disorder (PTSD).* Waterloo, Ontario: Institute Press.

Meyerson, D. A., Grant, K. E., Smith Carter, J., Kilmer, R. P. (2011) Posttraumatic growth among children and adolescents: A systematic review. *Clinical Psychology Review,* 31: 949–964.

Neimeyer, R. A. (2000) Narrative disruptions in the construction of self. In R. A. Neimeyer, J. D. Raskin (Eds.), *Constructions of disorder: Meaning making frameworks for psychotherapy* (pp. 207–241). Washington, DC: American Psychological Association.

Neimeyer, R. A. (2005) Widowhood, grief and the quest for meaning: A narrative perspective on resilience. In C. B. Wortman (Ed.), *Late life widowhood in the United States* (pp. 227–252). New York: Springer.

Neimeyer, R. A., Herrero, O., Botella, L. (2006) Chaos to coherence: Psychotherapeutic integration of traumatic loss. *Journal of Constructivist Psychology,* 19: 127–145.

Neimeyer, R. A., Levitt, H. (2001) Coping and coherence: A narrative perspective. In C. R. Snyder (Ed.), *Stress and coping* (pp. 47–67). New York: Oxford.

Nolen-Hoeksema, S., Morrow, J. (1991) A prospective study of depression and posttraumatic stress symptoms after a natural disaster: The 1989 Loma Prieta earthquake. *Journal of Personal and Social Psychology,* 61: 115–121.

Olema, D. K., Catani, C., Ertl, V., Saile, R., Neuner, F. (2014) The hidden effects of child maltreatment in a war region: Correlates of psychopathology in two generations living in Northern Uganda. *Journal of Traumatic Stress,* 27(1): 35–41.

Ong, A. D., Fulluer-Rowell, T. E., Bonanno, G. A. (2010) Prospective predictors of positive emotions following spousal loss. *Psychology and Aging,* 25: 631–640.

Ozer, E. J., Best, S. R., Lipsey, T. L., Weiss, D. S. (2003) Predictors of posttraumatic stress disorder and symptoms in adults: A meta-analysis. *Psychological Bulletin,* 129: 52–73.

Palmeiri, P. A, Danetti-Nisim, D., Galea, S., Johnson, R. J., Hobfoll, S. E. (2008) The psychological impact of the Israel-Hezbollah War on Jews and Arabs in Israel: The impact of risk and resilience factors. *Social Science & Medicine,* 67: 1208–1216.

Prati, G., Pietrantoni, L. (2009) Optimism, social support and coping strategies as factors contributing to posttraumatic growth: A meta-analysis. *Journal of Loss and Trauma,* 14: 364–388.

Roy-Byrne, P., Arguelles, L., Vitek, M. E., Goldberg, J., Keane, T. M., True, W. R., Pitman, R. K. (2004) Persistence and change of PTSD symptomatology: A longitudinal co-twin control analysis of the Vietnam Era Twin Registry. *Social Psychiatry and Psychiatric Epidemiology,* 39: 681–685.

Saegert, S., Thompson, J. P., Warren, M. R. (2001) *Social capital and poor communities.* New York: Russell Sage Foundation Publications.

Schnurr, P. P., Green, B. L. (2004) Understanding relationships among trauma, posttraumatic stress disorder and health outcomes. In P. P. Schnurr, B. L. Green (Eds.), *Trauma and health: Physical health consequences of exposure to extreme stress* (pp. 217–243). Washington, DC: American Psychological Association.

Sermpezis, C., Winter, D. A. (2009) Is trauma the product of over- or under-elaboration? A critique of the personal construct model of post-traumatic stress disorder. *Journal of Constructivist Psychology,* 22: 306–327.

Sewell. K. W. (1997) Post-traumatic stress: Towards a constructivist model of psychotherapy. In G. J. Neimeyer, R. A. Neimeyer (Eds.), *Advances in personal construct psychology* (Vol. 4, pp. 207–305). Greenwich, CT: JAI.

Sewell, K. W., Cromwell, R. L., Farrell-Higgins, J., Palmer, R., Ohlde, C., Patterson, T. W. (1996) Hierarchical elaboration in the conceptual structure of Vietnam veterans. *Journal of Constructivist Psychology,* 9: 79–96.

Sewell, K. W., Williams, A. M. (2000) Construing stress: A constructivist therapeutic approach to posttraumatic stress reactions. In R. A. Neimeyer (Ed.), *Meaning reconstruction and the experience of loss* (pp. 293–310). Washington, DC: American Psychological Association.

Shakespeare-Finch, J., Lurie-Beck, J. (2014) A meta-analytic clarification of the relationship between posttraumatic growth and symptoms of posttraumatic distress disorder. *Journal of Anxiety Disorders,* 28(2): 223–229.

Shephard, B. (2001) *A war of nerves: Soldiers and psychiatrists in the twentieth century*. Cambridge, MA: Harvard University Press.

Silverman, W. K., LaGreca, A. M. (2002) Children experiencing disasters: Definitions, reactions and predictors of outcomes. In A. M. LaGreca, W. K. Silverman, E. M. Vernberg, M. C. Roberts (Eds.), *Helping children cope with disasters and terrorism* (pp. 11–34). Washington, DC: American Psychological Association.

Space, L. G., Cromwell, R. L. (1980) Personal constructs among depressed patients. *Journal of Nervous and Mental Disease,* 168: 150–158.

Splevins, K., Cohen, K., Bowley, J., Joseph, S. (2010) Theories of posttraumatic growth: Cross cultural perspectives. *Journal of Loss and Trauma,* 15(3): 259–277.

Stein, M. B., Jang, K., Taylor, S., Vernon, P. A., Lively, W. J. (2002) Genetic and environmental influences on trauma exposure and posttraumatic stress disorder symptoms: A twin study. *American Journal of Psychiatry,* 159: 1675–1681.

Stiles, W. B., Osatuke, K., Glick, M., Mackay, H. C. (2004) Encounters between internal voices generate emotion. In H.J.M. Hermans, G. Dimaggio (Eds.), *The dialogical self in psychotherapy* (pp. 90–107). New York: Brunner Routledge.

Stokols, D. (1992) Establishing and maintaining healthy environments: Toward a social ecology of health promotion. *American Psychologist,* 47(1): 6–22.

Tedeschi, R. G., Calhoun, L. G. (1995) *Trauma and transformation: Growing in the aftermath of suffering*. Thousand Oaks, CA: Sage.

Tedeschi, R. G., Calhoun, L. G. (1996) The posttraumatic growth inventory: Measuring the positive legacy of trauma. *Journal of Traumatic Stress,* 9: 455–471.

Tedeschi, R. G., Calhoun, L. G. (2006) The foundations of posttraumatic growth: An expanded framework. In L. G. Calhoun, R. G. Tedeschi (Eds.), *Handbook of posttraumatic growth, research and practice* (pp. 3–23). Mahwah, NJ: Routledge.

Tennen, H., Affleck, G. (1999) Finding benefits in adversity. In C. R. Snyder (Ed.), *Coping: The psychology of what works* (pp. 279–304). New York: Oxford University Press.

Tucker, P., Pfefferbaum, B., Nixon, S. J., Dickson, W. (2000) Predictors of posttraumatic stress symptoms in Oklahoma City: Exposure, social support, peritraumatic response. *Journal of Behavioural Health Services and Research,* 27: 406–416.

Turner, S. W., Bowie, C., Dunn, G., Shapo, L., Yule, W. (2003) Mental health of Kosovan Albanian refugees in the UK. *The British Journal of Psychiatry,* 182: 444–448.

Ullman, J., Newcombe, M. (1999) I felt the earth move: A prospective study of the 1994 Northridge earthquake. In P. Cohen, C. Slomkowski, L. Robins (Eds.), *Historical and geographical influences on psychopathology* (pp. 217–246). Hillsdale, NJ: Erlbaum.

van der Kolk, B. A., van der Hart, O. (1991) The intrusive past: The flexibility of memory and the engraving of trauma. *American Imago,* 48: 425–454.

Walker, E. A., Keaton, W., Russo, J., Ciechanowski, P., Newman, E., Wagner, A. W. (2003) Health care costs associated with posttraumatic stress disorder symptoms in women. *Archive of General Psychiatry,* 60: 369–374.

Weems, C. F., Taylor, L. K., Cannon, M. F., Marino, R. C., Romano, D. M., Scott, B. G., Perry, A.M., Triplett, V. (2010) Posttraumatic stress, context, and the lingering effects of the Hurricane Katrina disaster among ethnic minority youth. *Journal of Abnormal Child Psychology,* 38: 49–56.

White, M., Epston, D. (1990) *Narrative means to therapeutic ends*. New York: Norton.

Wilson, J. P. (1994) The historical evolution of PTSD diagnostic criteria: From Freud to DSM-IV. *Journal of Traumatic Stress,* 7: 681–698.

Winter, D. A. (1992) *Personal construct psychology in clinical practice: Theory, research and applications*. London: Routledge.

Winter, D. A. (2003) Psychological disorder as imbalance. In F. Fransella (Ed.), *International handbook of personal construct psychology* (pp. 201–209). Chichester: Wiley.

Wolfe, J., Brown, P. J, Kelley, J. M. (1993) Reassessing war stress: Exposure and the Persian Gulf War. *Journal of Social Issues,* 49: 15–31.

Wortman, C. B., Silver, R. C. (1989) The myths of coping with loss. *Journal of Consulting and Clinical Psychology,* 57(3): 349–357.

Wright, M. O., Masten, A. S., Narayan, A. J. (2012) Resilience processes in development: Four waves of research on positive adaptation in the context of adversity. In S. Goldstein, R. B. Brooks (Eds.), *Handbook of resilience in children* (pp. 15–39). New York: Kluwer/ Academic Plenum.

# Chapter 3

# The people of Sierra Leone

Sierra Leone is an ethnically diverse nation of almost six million people, in a country that is similar in size to the Republic of Ireland. Having an outstanding natural harbour on the Atlantic coast, it was for many years a strategic location in maritime trading. Consequently, by the mid-eighteenth century, Sierra Leone had become well established in the trade route between Europe and the Americas. This role was to influence local traditions and the country's history significantly. Today, with over 50 years of independence from British colonial rule, Sierra Leone is one of the poorest countries in the world, despite its rich deposits of diamonds and iron ore.

## Ethnic groups

There are a total of 18 ethnic groups in Sierra Leone (United Nations Integrated Peacebuilding Office in Sierra Leone [UNIPSIL], 2014), each with a distinct version of the country's history. The largest group is the Mende, based in the southern and eastern provinces and embodying approximately one-third of the population. Approaching the same number are the Temne in the northern regions. The Limba, thought to be the oldest inhabitants of the country, are the third largest ethnic group, having been resident in the North for hundreds of years (Minorities at Risk [MAR], 2014). Other ethnic groups include the Kono in the East and the Koranko, Loko, Mandingo, Fula, Soso and Yalunka in the North. Along the coastal regions the Bullom and Sherbro groups predominate, alongside the much smaller groups of the Krim, Vai, Gola, and the Kissi, who reside further inland. The western area, including the capital, Freetown, has a more mixed population, which is predominantly Krio, together with a small number of Europeans and Lebanese. Despite this abundance of ethnic groups, Sierra Leone is unusual in the region for having a long history of ethnic, class and religious cordiality, with people often marrying between ethnicities (GlobalSecurity.org, 2014). However, in the second half of the twentieth century, it was an onerous task for these numerous and disparate communities to build a united and independent post-colonial nation (Annan, 1998).

The largest ethnic group, the Mende, have long resided in the southern and eastern regions of Sierra Leone. Linguistic evidence suggests that they migrated here from Guinea and Liberia during their role as hunters and raiders. Today, the Mende make up approximately one-third of the country's population. Their preponderance is thought to be due, in part, to their ability to assimilate well, an ability that has enabled them to play a great part in the history of West Africa (Alldridge, 1901). Their traditional structure utilizes a comparatively democratic system, electing Mende kings on merit and including women as rulers. Traditionally, the Mende believe in a supreme being, a sky god, and their ancestral spirits are highly revered. Humans, animals and objects are often thought to have a 'double' which has powers in the spirit world. A person's spirit may also leave his or her body during sleep to venture into the spirit world or, conversely, spirits may possess human form (Kelsall, 2009). The spirits are thought to act in either beneficial or harmful ways, depending on the gifts and sacrifices they receive from the living. In the post-colonial era, the Mende have been prominent in politics, vying for power and influence in long-standing disputes with the Temne.

Slightly smaller than the Mende population, the Temne ethnic group constitutes almost a third of Sierra Leone's population. They are predominantly located in the North of Sierra Leone, having originally migrated from Guinea. The Temne people are most easily identified by their unique language (MAR, 2014) and have a reputation as warriors, having had a history of disputes and domination. In their early establishment in Sierra Leone (in the early sixteenth century), they are thought to have forcibly displaced the Sherbro community from present-day Freetown. To be a leader of such warriors, Temne kings must successfully complete a series of training and tests. They are subsequently considered sacred and, as such, cannot be removed from office. Temne traditional belief describes space as being divided into four areas: humans/animals, demons, witches and ancestors. As documented by Littlejohn (1963), the latter three spaces are believed to be visible only to individuals who have 'two sets of eyes'.

The third largest ethnic group in Sierra Leone is the Limba. They are predominantly found in the northern half of the country. It has long been suggested that they are the oldest residents of Sierra Leone. This is evidenced by their linguistic peculiarities and the fact that, unlike all other groups, they lack a folklore explaining how they arrived in the country. The Limba speak numerous languages including, like the majority of the population, Krio. They primarily practice traditional animist religions, although there are also small numbers of Christians and Muslims (possibly the smallest proportion of Muslims of any ethnic group in Sierra Leone) (MAR, 2014). The Limba are mountainous people, who have strong beliefs in spirits known as 'krifi'. Their societal arrangements are somewhat less hierarchical than many other ethnic groups, and subjects may approach the chief directly, without the need for an intermediary.

In the East are the Kono people. They are thought to derive from a group that originally remained in the mountains during a wave of migration. Their folklore describes a salt shortage in Guinea, forcing their exodus to neigh-bouring Sierra Leone. Although currently less numerous than the Kono, the Mandingo (or Mandinka) are thought to be the group from which the Kono derived, the latter choosing to stay in the mountains whilst the Mandingo pushed on. Mandingos have long been recognized as effective traders, thanks primarily to their historic connections with Guinea. For two centuries the Mandingo were pivotal in the spread of Islam in Sierra Leone. However, from the early twentieth century, the Mandingo have been central actors in the diamond trade.

Believed to be related to the Mende population are the Loko, as demonstrated by their linguistic similarities. The Loko are thought to have been part of a sixteenth-century Mende settlement from which they were forcibly separated by Temne attacks. Their culture is greatly influenced by Temne customs, but it is the Temne who are believed to have traded heavily with the Portuguese in Loko slaves.

Whilst comprising less than 3 per cent of the population, the Creole com-munity has held a disproportionate political and economic power in Sierra Leone for many years. This is aptly demonstrated by its language, Krio, being the uniting *lingua franca* of the entire country. Creole influence derives from their origin as descendants of freed slaves, who settled in Freetown and soon assimilated Western culture and education. The new society in Freetown was created along Western lines but with African characteristics (Government of Sierra Leone, 1990). Education, language and religion were prioritized by the freed settlers, who saw Freetown as their city, the promised land. Although they initially intermarried with the indigenous population, they soon began to detach from the majority by acquiring British education and culture. As a result, Creoles occupied an inordinate number of government jobs, entailing higher status and greater financial reward. During the colonial period Creoles were thus very influential in the governmental and economic sectors. However, the British prevented them from dominating the political sphere (MAR, 2014). Traditionally, Creoles have regarded themselves as superior to the indigenous populations (Blyden, 1994), and vestiges of this status remain (Government of Sierra Leone, 1990).

Making up a small but significant portion of the Sierra Leonean population are the Lebanese. Despite a small presence of some 4,000, the Lebanese have maintained a disproportionate level of influence on trade in Sierra Leone. They first arrived at the end of the nineteenth century, having left Lebanon due to the loss of the lucrative silk market to cheaper Chinese and Japanese supplies. Leba-nese immigrants were initially beholden to British traders, but as they began to operate in rural areas where neither Europeans nor Creoles would travel, the Lebanese financial base grew. By 1966, 73 per cent of retail businesses were Lebanese-owned, and they remain heavily involved today, managing the major-ity of import-export to the country. More significantly, they still retain control of much of the diamond trade.

## Religious beliefs and social structures

Religious beliefs can significantly influence an individual's outlook. Consistent with many other African countries, the majority of the population of Sierra Leone believes in a close relationship between the visible (human) and invisible (spiritual) worlds. As Kelsall (2009) describes, the two worlds are thought to be constantly interacting, with beings from one world routinely intervening on the plane of the other. Many humans and some ordinary objects can possess supernatural powers. In fact, an individual's personal and political power is often thought to rely heavily on relationships with the spirits (Ellis & ter Haar, 2004). Ancestral spirits are of particular salience. They are unpredictable in their presentation as forces of good or evil, and thus offerings are constantly provided. Common to most indigenous religions in Sierra Leone is the belief in a supreme being. There is also a strong belief in the power of medicines to control the human world. Medicines can be used to facilitate contact between humans and spirits for diverse purposes (Bellman, 1984), from protecting property to facilitating love affairs or obtaining political power.

With regard to theist religions, Conteh (2011) describes Sierra Leoneans as believing that God has ultimate responsibility and overview for all that happens in the world. As a result, Sierra Leoneans may appear a somewhat resigned people. "Things change but seldom because of anything we do" (quoted in Jackson, 2004, p. 9). This is frequently related to religious belief: "God is great. He rewards our efforts. . . . Now I am only living by God." (Jackson, 2004, pp. 126 & 176). Historically a religiously tolerant society, Sierra Leone is primarily a Muslim country (60%), with the remainder of the population split between Christianity (20%) and animism (20%). In reality there is a large degree of assimilation and continued practice of animist religions in conjunction with both Islam and Christianity. For example, Christian individuals may both pray to God and visit an animist elder to address the same issue. Belief in the magic powers associated with animist religions should not be underestimated in Sierra Leone.

Ethnicity brings with it the beneficial attributes of kinship, language, history, culture and, moreover, identity. It defines the individual as an ethnic subject whose identity is rooted in his or her own particular explanation of events (Kandeh, 1992). In Sierra Leone, well-structured hierarchies exist within these ethnicities. Although variations exist, in general a paramount chief (elected or inherited depending on ethnicity) maintains ultimate respect and authority. In some groups, such as the Mende, the chief can be female or male and, also, dependent on the group, may be addressed either directly or through numerous intermediaries. In the Koranko ethnic group, a simple hierarchy is well established; people are superior to animals, first born are superior to second born, adults are superior to children, husbands to wives, and so on. This is the generally accepted lineage, although there can be some blurring of the lines. For example, displays of moral courage may elevate a person beyond a given social position (Jackson, 2004). In addition, rather than the individuality observed in the Western world, people in traditional African societies focus their lives around the extended family and the kinship group (Blyden, 1994). Group interests are of paramount concern and override those of the individual. In other words, more emphasis is placed on society than on the self (Jackson, 2004). The strong ethnic communities resulting from this approach reinforce the importance of kinship bonds and support weaker individuals. Throughout Sierra Leone's history, these ethnic chiefdoms and strong communities have been of paramount importance. They have consequently been closely linked with the politics of the country.

For as long as the indigenous populations have been present in Sierra Leone, there have been secret societies. These gender-specific organizations nurture the traditions and values of the community and develop extremely strong bonds between members. In earlier times, this would have involved three years of a child's life in 'bush school'. However, with the establishment of Western-style education, the extended bush learning process has declined but initiation into a society remains. For girls, this involves preparing them for marriage and motherhood. Once their initiation is complete they are considered to have made the transition to womanhood. Most commonly, this is at the time of the girls' first menstruation. The incidence of female genital mutilation (FGM) in initiation rites, with its consequential and enduring pain, is an area of grave concern, particularly as Sierra Leone has one of the highest rates of FGM in the world (UNICEF, 2014). The initiation ceremony for boys is group-based, where they learn about hunting, ethics, politics and social and individual responsibilities. They are trained in the traditions of the society and to obey the authority of elders. The boys are introduced to the practice of magic and, in a generally less injurious experience than the girls, are circumcised. Membership in a secret society is seen as essential for both men and women and for the cohesion and preservation of their communities. An example of this is the widespread secret society *Poro*, which mobilized multiple ethnic groups in the resistance which, as we shall see, emerged to the Hut Tax in 1898.

## History prior to the civil war

The history of Sierra Leone has long been a turbulent one, with numerous chronicles of invasion, slavery and civil war. Like many African populations, the peoples of Sierra Leone have an extended history, with archaeological and linguistic evidence indicating that humans have populated the region for thousands of years. The coastal areas have been inhabited by communities such as the Temne for a considerable time, with populations from neighbouring regions later migrating inland. Sierra Leone is thus a country considered to have had 'waves of migration', with various ethnic groups arriving at different times. Whilst these groups had strong tribal identities and some rivalries, they remained open to outsiders. Individuals intermarried and some groups, such as the Limba, even appointed outsiders as tribal chiefs. Consequently, Sierra Leone is not victim to the same degree of interethnic animosity as that observed in many other African states.

After many years of intra-African migration, it was not until the fifteenth century that the term Sierra Leone first became associated with the region. The Portuguese sailor Pedro da Cintra named the area *Serra Lyoa* – Lion Mountains – after the view of the mountainous peninsula from his ship. Trading with the Portuguese involved the exchange of gold and ivory for swords and utensils. Initially, this progressed well. However, with the demand for labour for plantations in the Americas, it soon became apparent that human beings were a far more valuable commodity. Also wishing to benefit fully from the highly profitable slave trade, British, Dutch and other European nations followed the Portuguese to the region. At the outset, slavery is thought to have involved kidnapping, as it was not then a tradition within the peoples of Sierra Leone (Rodney, 1972). However, it subsequently progressed to a highly lucrative trade, with countless individuals supplied by local chiefs. Many prisoners of war were sold to tribal leaders together with those accused of witchcraft or criminal activity. African traders received European goods, such as arms and brandy, in return for a seemingly inexhaustible supply of slaves. In 1672, a fort was established on Bunce Island by the British Royal African Company. This became a prime site of slave transportation (UNIPSIL, 2014). Located 20 miles from Freetown, it acted as a processing centre for slaves captured inland. They were brought to the castle and kept in harrowing conditions. Many did not make it onto the boats but died on the island. In total, it is believed that between 1668 and 1807 over 50,000 individuals sailed from this single point.

With increasing resistance from the enslaved and protests from those who had escaped, the many horrors of the slave trade eventually became apparent to a wider audience, and efforts began to abolish the practice. With the support of individuals such as the British member of Parliament William Wilberforce, the slave trade was outlawed in 1807, with slavery itself finally legally abolished in 1833.

In 1787, before the necessary acts of parliament were passed, the nascent British abolitionist movement established a settlement in Sierra Leone known as the 'Province of Freedom' (later to become Freetown). Freed slaves sailed first from London and later from Nova Scotia to settle as free people. Any slave reaching the soil of Freetown was entitled to claim their freedom, and by 1792, 1,200 freed slaves had joined the original settlers. Freetown became a British Crown Colony in 1808. As it was the principal centre for the suppression of the slave trade, it was equipped with a newly established naval base to intercept any illicit slave ships. The success of these activities was somewhat mixed, with documentation indicating that an illicit trade in slaves continued for several years (Macaulay, 1831). However, by this time the British were firmly established in Sierra Leone, and Freetown served as the seat of government for several British colonies in West Africa. Initially, British administration in Sierra Leone was limited to the colony of Freetown, a situation the British wished to maintain due to the expense of administering a colony that was not yet profitable and where, by 1855, over 50,000 freed slaves had settled.

Over the remainder of the nineteenth century, the British obtained influence over the coast and hinterland near Freetown, mostly without providing effective (expensive) administration. At the same time, the French were expanding their dominance in Africa and encroaching towards Freetown. In response, the regions not considered to be under French or Liberian influence were proclaimed a British protectorate in 1896 (Hargreaves, 1956). The sociopolitical organization of the protectorate lands was exclusively tribal at the time. The region was home to over a hundred individual chiefdoms and approximately fourteen tribal groups. The establishment of the British protectorate implied arbitrary political unification across these groups. Despite a British desire to enhance its 'spheres of influence' throughout the interior, by 1890 no truly sympathetic contact with Sierra Leonean society had been established. Thus there were tensions existing long before British administrative policies put them under breaking strain.

In 1898, to raise revenue for developing the region, the British imposed what they saw as a just and essential five shilling tax on every home. In the North, resistance to the tax from Temne chiefs developed into open warfare, and Mende and Sherbro chiefs in the South subsequently joined this brutal nine-month uprising. Known as the Hut Tax War, it was the first large-scale war in Sierra Leone. The British interpretation of the rebellion was that the Hut Tax and other actions of the administration were unacceptable to the indigenous population. They thought that the local population was deliberately rejecting progress, wanting 'a reversion to the old order of things such as fetish customs, slave-dealing and raiding' (Cardew, 1898, as quoted in Hargreaves [1956], p. 57). Historians such as Hargreaves (1956) suggest that rather than a sudden resistance to an administrative malpractice, it was in fact the reaction of a conservative and static community to several years of colonial rule. The population of the protectorate was not familiar with a system of taxation, where payment to a centralized state contributes towards services provided. Moreover, the combination of the British administration charging people for their own homes together with rumours that they were to start appropriating land led to foreboding in the minds of the indigenous communities. The focus of their alarm lay not only with the British presence but also with the Creoles, due to their continued alignment with the colonizing nation. Many Creoles were attacked and killed, thus further obstructing the development of any sense of common nationhood between Creole and indigenous ethnicities for a considerable number of years. The British sent in troops to combat the uprising. Hundreds were killed, but the tax was ultimately retained. Chiefs who successfully collected the tax were often 'honoured' with a proportion of it. It could be suggested that the British were thus responsible for creating a culture of political corruption in Sierra Leone.

The division between the Creole and the ethnic groups of the protectorate population continued from the end of the nineteenth century until independence. During this time, Creoles rejected political equality, considering the indigenous groups savage and barbarian (Blyden, 1994). Unsurprisingly, the protectorate communities took exception to Creole political dominance and their assertion of superiority. Reinforcing this divide was the British law determining that Creoles were British subjects whilst individuals from the interior were merely considered British protected persons. This political, administrative and legal dualism strongly influenced the ethnoregional conflicts during the consolidation (1900–1940) and terminal (1940–1961) phases of colonial rule (Kandeh, 1992).

Creole dominance began to wane at the dawn of the twentieth century as the demographics of Freetown began to change. This was occurring on two levels. First, there was urbanization. Between 1891 and 1911, the composition of Freetown residents transformed from 58 per cent Creole, 40 per cent protectorate ethnic groups to 36 per cent Creole, 61 per cent protectorate. Creoles generally felt threatened by this influx into what they considered to be exclusively their city, their promised land (Kandeh, 1992). A defining moment in the decline of Creole dominance was the Tribal Administration (Freetown) Act of 1905. In order to regulate and control the different protectorate groups present in Freetown, the British recognized tribal headmen as being involved in the well-being of their members in Freetown. In effect, the tribal chiefs acted as intermediaries in the administration's attempts to obtain social order (Banton, 1957). As a result, the tribal heads in Freetown contributed to competition between ethnicities, advancing the British policy of divide and rule, thus enabling the British to wield power more easily in the absence of a united population.

The second factor influencing the wane of Creole dominance was the influx of Europeans and Lebanese to Freetown. Newly arriving Europeans began to establish themselves at higher-altitude hill stations to avoid the fatality of malaria. This enabled the numbers of Europeans in Freetown to swell, with the majority filling government positions previously held by Creoles. At the same time, Lebanese were replacing Creole merchants as commercial intermediaries. This somewhat usurped the long-established Creole-British relationship, further adding to the demise of Creole influence.

In World War I, 17,000 Sierra Leoneans were drafted to fight for the British. On their return, dissatisfaction with low wages was demonstrated by the railway strike of 1919. Opposition to British governance continued to grow, and in 1924 a new constitution was drawn up allowing indigenous groups to have political representation in Freetown. This had previously only been available to the Creole and British, but new political organizations had come into being, the most prominent reflecting the deeply embedded division between the Creole and indigenous populations. The Sierra Leone branch of the National Congress of British West Africa (NCBWA) was exclusively Creole, whilst the Committee of Educated Aborigines (CEA) was founded by indigenous groups in 1922. At this time, the disparities existing between Freetown and the interior were stark. The population of Freetown (where the majority of Creoles lived) stood at 60,000, compared to 2 million in the protectorate. In addition, the two areas differed in political organization and land rights. Whilst the 1905 act had established tribal headmen within Freetown, the protectorate had direct rule. Land in Freetown could be bought and sold on an open market whilst that in the protectorate was held in perpetuity for the populace. In an attempt to unify the populations, the Stevenson Constitution of 1947 further widened political representation. Once again, the Creoles protested against this expansion, but their progressive decline towards political marginalization could not be halted, and activities of other, numerically superior, groups began to dominate.

The mid-twentieth century saw the founding of two significant parties, again reflecting the Creole and indigenous groups division: the National Council for Sierra Leone (NCSL, Creole) and the Sierra Leone Peoples' Party (SLPP, protectorate). The SLPP was in fact formed predominantly from the Mende population, with the notable exception of future president Siaka Stevens, who was from the North. With the move towards independence starting to take shape, a framework for decolonization was drawn up in a new constitution in 1951. In the corresponding elections, the SLPP's success was overwhelming (which further marginalized the Creole population). As a result, only SLPP members were selected by the British to sit on the Executive Council. In 1953, in a further move to autonomy, ministerial responsibility was transferred to local representatives and SLPP leader Milton Margai was appointed chief minister. After several years, Margai became the first prime minister of Sierra Leone and oversaw the lead-up to its independence in 1961. But this was not before a breakaway party was formed by Milton's half brother, Albert Margai, with Siaka Stevens. This was the All People's Congress (APC). Stevens was eager to hold an election prior to independence to demonstrate that a viable alternative existed to the SLPP. However, Milton Margai responded by declaring a state of emergency and imprisoning all SLPP leaders.

On 27 April 1961, Sierra Leone was granted independence from Great Britain under its first prime minister, SLPP leader and Mende, Milton Margai. Although Mende and Temne groups had previously united in a common resentment of the Creoles, after independence the two groups battled for power. Allies had become adversaries. Milton Margai reacted to the concerns of the Temne by appointing them in ministerial positions. However, it was not sufficient to prevent them creating a potent opposition to the SLPP. The APC, now solely under Stevens, was perceived by many Temne and others as the party to end elite Mende dominance and to facilitate Temne social emancipation. Unsurprisingly, in the elections of 1967, the APC and its populist rhetoric (a party for the masses as opposed to the privileged) won a landslide victory. The reality is that whilst the SLPP was criticized for being Mende-dominated, the APC was equally Temne-dominated, and this time the resentment was from the Mende.

The APC were initially welcomed as an idealistic government, but allegations of corruption soon surfaced as Stevens revealed an inclination towards dictatorship. In 1973, all opposition candidates withdrew from the election due to the threat of violence. Finally, in 1978, the APC declared Sierra Leone a one-party state. Stevens justified this by declaring that it would put an end to conflicts and resentments between the country's different ethnic groups. In effect, it actually served to create increasingly defined cultural identities and divisions. Rancid corruption and misjudged spending accompanied the lack of democracy, and the country spiraled into worsening poverty. Education and enterprise were eroded. Diamond trading was rerouted via APC strongholds, and Stevens took personal responsibility for the US$300 million per annum industry. He appointed personal friend Jamil Mohammed Khalil, a Lebanese trader, to manage the business. According to the then finance minister, a reported US$160 million was lost per year to diamond smuggling. Moreover, legally exported diamonds dropped from over 2 million carats in 1970 to a mere 48,000 carats in 1988 (Smillie, Gabrie & Hazleton, 2000), and the country's finances continued to deteriorate.

In 1985, after over 14 years in office, Stevens handed the presidency to his chosen successor, Joseph Saidu Momoh. Once again, idealist rhetoric was proclaimed, with Momoh stating that he would challenge diamond smuggling and tax evasion. Tragically, no change occurred, and despite presiding over a report recommending the reestablishment of a multiparty system, the APC remained the sole party in Sierra Leone at the outbreak of the long and bloody civil war in 1991.

## Conclusions

In contemplating responses to adversity, such as those faced in the civil war of Sierra Leone, it is imperative that cultural considerations are made central (Kleber, Figley & Gersons, 1995; Segall, Lonner & Berry, 1998). People's assumptions, their ability to modify these in adversity, and their social support are all factors affected by culture (McMillen, 2004). Bracken (1998) argues that Western psychology heavily exports cognitivism, the commitment to reliving the trauma in order to acquire cognitive mastery to eliminate the fear response. However, this is often irrelevant in non-Western societies where there is a strong kindred, cultural and spiritual response. Interventions should accommodate this. According to Herman (1992), common to the recovery from trauma of all cultures is the requirement to reconstruct meaning, rebuild hope and regain control. The imposition of a decontextualized and culturally ignorant approach would at the very least limit healing and at worst confound the trauma.

Stress and trauma should be understood within the particular context of an individual's belief systems, spiritual practices and the unique event itself. This is underlined by the American Psychological Association (2010), which notes in its ethical standards that faith traditions should be recognized in the provision of ethical treatment. It also recognizes (American Psychological Association, 2013) that religious institutions can be important sources of support for trauma survivors. However, religious and spiritual beliefs may not be readily disclosed to outsiders (Peddle, Monteiro, Guluma & Macaulay, 1999), and psychologists must therefore approach with care. Ultimately, any approach must respect the view of the world held by that person. It is also important not to decontextualize and impose an external society's perception of what constitutes a traumatic event. For example, Peddle et al. (1999) describe a woman in Sierra Leone telling of how she and her family had been displaced during the war. Her father died during their evacuation and, due to the necessity to move on quickly, did not receive a proper funeral, simply a shallow burial. To most outsiders, the death of her father would appear to be the cause of trauma. In fact, the woman was accepting of the loss; what had traumatized her was the inability to give her father a proper burial and the significance of this in terms of her cultural traditions and beliefs.

The scale of psychological needs is extremely apparent in situations of armed conflict (Wessels, 1998), which are currently a major cause of trauma in Africa. The impact of conflict does not rest solely with the individual. Rather, it is firmly tied to the devastation of families and whole communities (Reichenberg & Friedman, 1996). The majority of fatalities in contemporary conflicts are civilians. Weapons of war include rape and mutilation, often undertaken by those previously living as neighbours. Therefore, community-based approaches, particularly those that consider traditional healing, should be encouraged (Hudnall-Stamm, Stamm, Hudnall & Higson-Smith, 2004). Correspondingly, individualistic responses may be completely inappropriate and unsuccessful. Furthermore, in the aftermath of war, psychologists may delve straight to psychological issues when more immediate problems, such as food security, must first be addressed (consistent with Maslow's hierarchy of needs hypothesis), and clinicians should remain mindful of the fact that Western concepts and methods are not necessarily appropriate or effective in all cultural contexts.

Later chapters in this book will demonstrate the resilience of the people of Sierra Leone, their powerful ability to promote healing and rebuild lives, a capacity which should be harnessed to maximum effect.

## References

Alldridge, T. J. (1901) *The Sherbro and its hinterland: An introduction to the area.* New York: Macmillan.

American Psychological Association (2010) *Ethical principles of psychologists and code of conduct (2002, Amended June 1, 2010).* Available at: http://www.apa.org/ethics/code/index.aspx [Accessed 1 July 2014].

American Psychological Association (2013) *Protecting our children from abuse and neglect.* Available at: http://www.apa.org/pi/families/resources/abuse.aspx [Accessed 1 July 2014].

Annan, K. (1998) *The causes of conflict and the promotion of durable peace and sustainable development in Africa.* (Report of the Secretary-General to the United Nations Security Council A/52/871-S/1998/318). New York: United Nations.

Banton, M. (1957) *West African city.* London: Oxford University Press.

Bellman, B. L. (1984) *The language of secrecy: Symbols and metaphor in Poro ritual.* New Brunswick, NJ: Rutgers University Press.

Blyden, E. W. (1994) *African life and customs*. Baltimore, MD: Black Classic Press.

Bracken, P. J. (1998) *Rethinking the trauma of war*. London: Free Association Press.

Cardew to Chamberlain, Confidential, 28 May 1898. As quoted in Hargreaves, J. D. (1956) The establishment of the Sierra Leone Protectorate and the insurrection of 1898. *Cambridge Historical Journal,* 12 (1): 56–80.

Conteh, S. (2011) *Major religions of Sierra Leone*. Canada: Xlibris.

Ellis, S., ter Haar, G. (2004) *Worlds of power: Religious thought and political practice in Africa*. London: Hurst.

GlobalSecurity.org (2014) *Sierra Leone*. Available at: http://www.globalsecurity.org [Accessed 23 July 2014].

Government of Sierra Leone (1990) *Area handbook for Sierra Leone*. Freetown, Sierra Leone: Ministry of Education.

Hargreaves, J. D. (1956) The establishment of the Sierra Leone Protectorate and the insurrection of 1898. *Cambridge Historical Journal,* 12 (1): 56–80.

Herman, J. (1992) *Trauma and recovery*. New York: HarperCollins.

Hudnall-Stamm, B., Stamm, H. E., Hudnall, A. C., Higson-Smith, C. (2004) Considering a theory of cultural trauma and loss. *Journal of Trauma and Loss: International Perspectives on Stress and Coping,* 9 (1): 89–111.

Jackson, M. (2004) *In Sierra Leone*. Durham, NC, & London: Duke University Press.

Kandeh, J. D. (1992) Politicization of ethnic identities in Sierra Leone. *African Studies Review,* 35(1): 81–99.

Kelsall, T. (2009) *Culture under cross-examination: International justice and the Special Court for Sierra Leone*. Cambridge: Cambridge University Press.

Kleber, R., Figley, C. R., Gersons, B. (Eds.) (1995) *Beyond trauma*. New York: Plenum.

Littlejohn, J. (1963) Temne space. *Anthropological Quarterly,* 36(1): 1–17.

Macaulay, Z. (1831) *Antislavery Monthly Report Volume 3*. London: Hatchard.

McMillen, J. (2004) Posttraumatic growth: What's it all about? *Psychological Inquiry,* 15: 48–52.

Minorities at Risk (MAR) (2014) *Assessments for Creole, Limba, Mende, Temne in Sierra Leone*. Available at: http://www.cidcm.umd.edu/mar/assessment.asp?groupld=45102 [Accessed 24 July 2014].

Peddle, N., Monteiro, C., Guluma, V., Macaulay, T. (1999) Trauma, loss and resilience in Africa: A psychosocial community based approach to culturally sensitive healing. In K. Nader, N. Dubrow, B. H. Stamm (Eds.), *Honoring differences, cultural issues in the treatment of trauma and loss* (pp. 1–19). London: Brunner/Mazel.

Reichenberg, D., Friedman S. (1996) Traumatized children. Healing the invisible wounds of war: A rights approach. In Y. Danieli, N. S. Rodley, L. Weisath (Eds.), *International responses to traumatic stress* (pp. 307–326). Amityville, NY: Baywood.

Rodney, W. (1972) *How Europe underdeveloped Africa*. London: Bogle-L'Ouverture Publications.

Segall, M. H., Lonner, W. J., Berry, J. W. (1998) Cross-cultural psychology as a scholarly discipline: On the flowering of culture in behavioural research. *American Psychologist,* 53(10): 1101–1110.

Smillie, I., Gabrie, N., Hazleton, R. (2000) *The diamond of the matter: Sierra Leone, diamonds and human security*. Ottawa: Partnership Africa-Canada.

UNICEF (2014) *UNICEF Data: Monitoring the situation of children and women*. Available at: http://data.unicef.org/child-protection/fgmc [Accessed 6 September 2014].

United Nations Integrated Peacebuilding Office in Sierra Leone (UNIPSIL) (2014) Available at: http://unipsil.unmissions.org [Accessed 25 June 2014].

Wessels, M. G. (1998) The changing nature of armed conflict and its implications for children: the Graca Machel/UN study. *Peace and Conflict: Journal of Peace Psychology,* 4(4): 321–334.

# Chapter 4

# Eleven years of civil war and eleven years of recovery

## Eleven years of civil war

Sierra Leone's 11-year civil war began in March 1991 between the government and Sierra Leonean dissidents. Under Siaka Stevens, whose rule from 1968 to 1985 was called 'the seventeen-year plague of locusts' (Hirsch, 2001, p. 29), all levels of state administration had been affected, and for years to come (Kandeh, 2002). The corruption under both Stevens and General Joseph Momoh '. . . destroyed the enterprise of the people and their will to be governed' (Zack-Williams, 1999, p. 144), which in turn further encouraged rebellion and war.

Thus the groundwork was laid, and it was easy to engage political thugs, Liberians, and mercenaries from Burkina Faso and Libya, who were all led by Foday Saybana Sankoh (Adebajo, 2002; Hirsch, 2001; Rosen, 2005). Sankoh was disgruntled with the political system and the effects of patrimonial rule. His dissatisfaction was reinforced in his relationship with Liberian president Charles Taylor (Abraham, 2001). Taylor had a vested interest in a successful revolt against the Sierra Leonean government: his continued search for resources, such as control of Sierra Leone's diamond mines, and a desire for revenge against the government (Goins, 2015).

In March 1991, Sankoh organized the Revolutionary United Front (RUF), with youth making up a large part of this group (Peters, 2006; Richards, 1996; Rosen, 2005).[1] Sankoh and the RUF purportedly wanted to restore democracy, exposing and removing the 'corrupt regime from power' (Jackson, 2004, p. 142). 'Footpaths to Democracy: Toward a New Sierra Leone' was the ethos of the RUF. People should take up arms '. . . in order to take back their power and use this power to create wealth for themselves and generations to come . . .' (RUF, 1995).

The RUF launched a campaign against the government by attacking villages, farmers, and current holders of the diamond mines in the south and southeast regions of the country (Goins, 2015). The alliance between Sankoh and Taylor fuelled the conflict. Weapons came through trade, primarily of diamonds, across the Liberian border (Campbell, 2002). The RUF's tactics were horrendous, including child and adult abductions, beatings, torture, murder, mutilation, violent rituals, rape, arson and looting, which accelerated as the war proceeded and increasingly alienated the rural population (Abraham, 2001; Adebajo, 2002; Appadurai, 1999; Bangura, 1997; Campbell, 2002; Forna, 2002; Gbla, 2003; Lyon, 2004; McKay & Mazurana, 2004; PHR, 2003; Weissman, 2003). Then Sierra Leonean president Joseph Saidu Momoh, in his attempt to overcome this rebellion, rallied existing government troops and sought to recruit new ones.

Unfortunately, the government's instability increased as the war progressed, its small, ineffectual army ill equipped to defend the country against the invading RUF (Rosen, 2005). Two coups later, Alhaji Ahmed Tejan Kabbah, a former UN official and leader of the Sierra Leone People's Party (SLPP), was chosen as president. He won with 72 per cent of the votes in a free election, but not without severe suffering by the civilian population (Abraham, 2001; Adebajo, 2002; Kandeh, 2003). The rebels and government army protested violently by indiscriminately amputating the hands or legs of countless people, including children, to prevent or exact punishment for voting (Abraham, 2001).

A South African military outfit, Executive Outcomes (EO), had successfully combatted the RUF to the point of bringing them to negotiations in Abidjan, Côte d'Ivoire, when Kabbah was in power (Chege, 2002). Kabbah and Sankoh signed the Abidjan Peace Agreement, the first of the peace agreements, in November 1996 (Hirsch, 2001). However, conditional to the ceasefire was EO withdrawing and all foreign troops repatriating, which left Sierra Leone vulnerable to further attack (Abraham, 2001; Adebajo, 2002; Chege, 2002). With EO gone, the RUF allied with the national army (the Sierra Leone Army or SLA). In May 1997, they staged a coup (Adebajo, 2002; Hirsch, 2001). Kabbah fled to Guinea until 1998, when he was reinstated, and a junta between the newly formed Armed Forces Revolutionary Council (AFRC) and the RUF was formed (Goins, 2015). There were further massacres of civilians, especially in the capital (Glover, 1999). Major Johnny Paul Koroma became the head of the AFRC.

In the beginning of 1998, the Economic Community of West African States Cease-Fire Monitoring Group (ECOMOG) overcame the AFRC/RUF alliance. Kabbah was reinstated as president in March of that year. Sankoh was captured, imprisoned and sentenced (Hirsch, 2001). Nevertheless, by January 1999, the RUF controlled 80 per cent of the country (Shepler, 2005, p. 47). On January 6, 1999, the RUF launched one of its bloodiest campaigns in Freetown, marking it as the day most Freetown Sierra Leoneans will never forget (Goins, 2015). After two months of fighting, the ECOMOG and civil defence forces (CDFs) finally drove RUF soldiers out from the city. The RUF took several thousand children and adults with them.

All armed groups were guilty of human rights violations, including torture, rape, murder, abductions, destruction of property, looting and/or transgressing national as well as international law (Goins, 2015; Govier, 2006; HRW, 1999; Mazurana & Carlson, 2004; Rosen, 2005; Zack-Williams, 2001). All armed groups earned their reputations, though some were more destructive. The RUF, the most offensive of these armed groups, came to be emblematic of the others who committed equally offensive acts (Goins, 2015).

When the Lomé Peace Agreement[2] was signed in July 1999, the UN Security Council said, '(it is) . . . a historic turning point for all Sierra Leone and its people' (Hirsch, 2001, p. 126). The RUF received blanket amnesty for atrocities committed against the civilian population from March 1991 to July 1999, as well as a platform to become a legitimate political party (Abraham, 2001; Hirsch, 2001). All parties (including the RUF, AFRC, SLA, civil defence forces – or CDFs – and the government) were to benefit from a programme of disarmament, demobilization and reintegration (DDR) of all combatants (Article XVI), and a more specific reference to child combatants (Article XXX). The UN Assistance Mission in Sierra Leone (UNAMSIL) brought, albeit temporary, stability to the country and to Freetown in particular by bringing in 6,000 peacekeeping troops. Nevertheless, in May 2000, the RUF attacked Freetown again. Fighting between government forces and armed groups continued late into 2001, but the presence of, by this time, a record 18,500-strong peacekeeping force seemed to be what was needed to stop the momentum of the war and finally bring it to an end.[3]

On 18 January 2002, the day after one of us (Stephanie Goins) arrived in the country for her fieldwork, the war was officially declared over. Civilian casualties numbered a minimum of 70,000, but this is impossible to document (Chege, 2002). Tens of thousands were killed (Rosen, 2005). Amputees officially numbered 770, reflecting the government's caseload, but Chege claims that thousands suffered from amputations. The number of displaced children was estimated at 1.8 million (Mawson, Dodd & Hilary, 2000). During the war more than a third of the population was displaced (Rosen, 2005); this included 750,000 who were internally displaced. As of 2004, over half had returned to their places of origin, some with government assistance and some without. At the close of 2000, nearly 400,000 Sierra Leoneans were refugees and asylum seekers. In 2003, the overall number of refugees had reduced to 71,000. As of 2004, Sierra Leone was also hosting 70,000 refugees from Liberia, putting further strain on an already depleted government.[4]

### Suggested causes for the war

Since the early 1960s, Sierra Leone has been subjected to corrupt governments, insurgencies and military coups, and such economic mismanagement and instability that it is easy to see why it plummeted to the ranking of least developed nation in the countries listed by the United Nations Development Programme (UNDP), though this has fluctuated over the years. As to the origins or causes of the war, it has been suggested that poor governance, economic injustice, corruption, greed, elitism, a crisis of youth, the disintegration of the family and general apathetic attitudes of Sierra Leoneans all contributed.

Poor governance contributed overall to the collapse of the state and its education and social services (Abraham, 2001; Chege, 2002; Hirsch, 2001; Jackson, 2004; Keen, 2005; Reno, 1995; TRC, 2004). Economic injustice, corruption, patrimonial rule and elitism also contributed (Baksh-Soodeen & Etchart, 2001; Bangura, 1997; Gberie, 2004; Glover, 1999; Govier, 2006; Kandeh, 2002; Noyes, 2003; Olonisakin, 2000; Zack-Williams, 1999). People were either 'coerced into silence or forced into exile. The latter group constitutes the vanguard of the RUF' (Zack-Williams, 1999, p. 159). The brief history provided in the previous chapter supports any of these suggested causes of war.

Since the ending of the war, academics and Sierra Leone nationals have cited the control over one of the country's most valuable resources, diamonds, as the main contributor (Baker & May, 2004; Campbell, 2002; Goins, 2015). While it may be true that the war was fought for several years without major diamond income, diamonds certainly fuelled the war (Davies, 2002; Peters, 2006). 'The greed of the big ones (those in power, such as elders and chiefs) is the real problem', according to Shepler (2005, p. 107). According to interviewees, greed was a huge factor for participation in an armed group.

Others refer to globalization, which fuelled the 'crisis of youth' (Appadurai, 1999; Bangura, 1997; Kandeh, 2002; Richards, 1996; Rosen, 2005). Youth were disenfranchised, educationally disadvantaged, fighting against the state corruption and injustice, and fighting for education and jobs (Goins, 2015; Peters, 2006; Richards, 1996; Rosen, 2005). When youth are not cared for by the state, inevitably they lose hope and may turn to banditry and thuggery (Kandeh, 2002).

According to Peters and Richards (1998), the RUF was a revolutionary movement comprised of excluded intellectuals. They rebelled against corrupt governance and oppression. However, others do not believe this to be the case. Rather, the RUF lacked 'the organisational and ideological characteristics and discipline of revolutionary movements as they are known' (Abraham, 2001, p. 207), and their barbaric tactics were further proof of that (Abdullah, 1997; Abdullah & Muana, 1998; Bangura, 1997). Goins (2015) and Shepler (2005) found that most Sierra Leoneans would agree with Bangura. 'They (the RUF) may have begun with a core group of politically oriented revolutionaries, but their activities soon devolved into terror and banditry' (Shepler, 2005, p. 139).

Because of the many ethnic groups in Sierra Leone, it was repeatedly suggested that the war was caused by ethnic tension and competition. However, this supposition is largely refuted by several sources, including interviewees, who said the war was not ethnically based (Goins, 2015). 'Sierra Leone did not experience the ethnic fratricide that is often blamed for state collapse in Africa before or after independence' (Chege, 2002, p. 148). 'There is no centuries-old ethnic conflict fuelling the bloodshed . . .' (Campbell, 2002, p. xxi). There may be some tension between ethnic groups in some respects (Davies, 2002), but most would agree that this was not the cause or origin of the war.[5]

Gberie (2004), citing a report from the Truth and Reconciliation Commission, says there is much overlap in the suggested causes:

> The report stresses that issues of bad governance, endemic corruption and poverty, disenchanted youth, a dictatorship that closed legitimate avenues of political expression, the dubious policies of the former colonial administration, uneven development in the country, capital punishment, a sclerotic elite, autocratic chiefs, a demented gerontocracy, patrimonial politics – all of these laid the grounds for the war which would have taken place even without the existence of diamonds in the country.[6]

Some link family and societal breakdown to the war. 'The emergence of child soldiers points to the transformation of society in Sierra Leone, in particular of the family' (Zack-Williams, 1999, p. 155). The increase of street children reflects this (Goins, 2015). Children feel they are not being properly cared for or listened to within their families and communities, which could have increased their vulnerability to participation. While the breakdown of the family is rarely noted as a cause for war, Sierra Leone nationals believe this to be the case (Goins, 2015).

Some have noted the general apathetic attitude that Sierra Leoneans have, which may be interpreted as 'a weapon of political protest' and 'stoic act of indifference' predominant in pre-war Sierra Leone (Sesay, 2004, p. 3). However, Shepler was told: 'We don't love ourselves; otherwise, one takes care for the other' (2005, p. 104). This circles back to family and society breakdown, a critical point to consider in the recovery process.

Sierra Leoneans generally see themselves as happy and relaxed people and could not believe the war had actually happened (Goins, 2015). They seemed to be confused by it. One interviewee said it was 'a complete breakdown of law and order' with nothing 'planned to put in its place'. Obviously, the war resulted in further breakdown of law and order. However, the pervasive attitude was an aversion and dislike for the war in the first place, which may have facilitated reintegration, rehabilitation and post-war recovery.

## Post-war recovery

As previously stated, the war was officially declared over in January 2002. In the post-war recovery process, the government of Sierra Leone utilized strategies articulated in two documents: the National Resettlement, Reconstruction and Rehabilitation (NRRR) document, and the National Disarmament, Demobilization and Reintegration (DDR) document. These two documents outlined programmes designed to disarm and demobilize ex-combatants and provide reintegration assistance through various means. The government established the National Committee for Disarmament, Demobilization and Reintegration (NCDDR) and the National Commission for Reconstruction, Resettlement and Rehabilitation, now known as the National Commission for Social Action (NaCSA), to oversee the implementation of these two programmes (Rugumamu & Gbla, 2003). Additionally, UN peacekeeping forces served to establish stability and security, which ensured peaceful democratic elections in 2002.

### Disarmament, demobilization and reintegration

Disarmament involves 'the collection, control and disposal of small arms, ammunitions, explosives and light and heavy weapons' (United Nations, 1999, p. 15). Disbanding armed groups, or demobilization, often included compensation or assistance for ex-combatants as they transitioned into civilian life. This process included '. . . counselling and training . . . tailored to . . . reflect political, social, economic and educational backgrounds' and benefit packages relevant to immediate needs, which could have included small-scale credit schemes (United Nations, 1999, p. 9; see also Rugumamu & Gbla, 2003). The reintegration phase involved actual integration into the community, either of origin or a new community. Reintegration incorporated the social and economic issues that concerned former soldiers (Goins, 2015).

The disarmament, demobilization and reintegration programme (DDRP) in Sierra Leone was funded by the World Bank, the British Department for International Development (DFID), and other donor governments and international non-governmental organizations (INGOs) (McKay & Mazurana, 2004; World Bank, 2002). Its establishment was supported through the Sierra Leone government as well as the United Nations Assistance Mission in Sierra Leone (UNAMSIL). Initiated in July 1998, the DDRP was interrupted by fighting. It picked up again in October 1999 until May 2000, but renewed hostilities put it to a halt again. One year later, in May 2001, the DDRP resumed operation until December 2003 (CSUCS, 2004).

Approximately 72,500 soldiers were disarmed and demobilized through the DDRP, with approximately 7,000 of these reported through the DDRP as being child soldiers.[7] However, the percentage of children involved in the beginning phase of the war was reported as high as 70 per cent (CSUCS, 2004). Thus, a large percentage of child soldiers, if they went through the DDRP, would have been disarmed as adults (Goins, 2015).

As with most DDR programmes, only those former soldiers who produced weapons for UNAMSIL were eligible for disarmament (World Bank, 2002). The 'one person, one gun' system yielded a cash reward of anywhere from 60,000 leones (at the time, US$30) to 600,000 leones (US$300). Later, the 'one person' system changed to group disarmament, in which commanders of armed groups provided a list of soldiers to be disarmed to UNAMSIL and the NCDDR.[8] In order to receive the benefits of those being disarmed as a group, former soldiers were required to demonstrate the use and disassembling of a gun. Thus, if a soldier served other functions in an armed group (and there were many such functions), s/he was not entitled to the DDR package.

Additionally, though it is well known that females killed just as males did, those officers overseeing the DDR process did not question the absence of females from a list (Goins, 2015). While this approach facilitated the disarmament process and reduced the recirculation of arms from across the Liberian border primarily, there were two basic problems: it allowed commanders to falsify the numbers of former soldiers and weaponry surrendered, and it ensured that former child soldiers, particularly girls, could be excluded (CSUCS, 2003; Lowicki & Pillsbury, 2002; McKay & Mazurana, 2004; World Bank, 2002).

During the disarmament phase, 42,330 weapons and 1.2 million pieces of ammunition were collected and destroyed (World Bank, 2002). However, the weapons most often used by the civil defence forces (CDFs) – hunting rifles, shotguns and machetes – were not counted (Goins, 2015; ICG, 2001). Thus, many former CDF soldiers who relied on these kinds of 'uncounted' weapons were not eligible for the DDR programme.

That said, whether a former child soldier actually had to turn in a weapon to qualify for the DDRP was questionable (McKay & Mazurana, 2004). Seven- to eleven-year-olds who did not produce a weapon but served in other capacities, who held a rank and/or were with an armed group more than six months were meant to be eligible for the DDRP (Williamson & Cripe, 2002). All former child soldiers were purportedly taken into interim care centres (ICCs) (Baker & May, 2004; Shepler, 2005). The 'weapons for cash' policy meant that children, and particularly female former soldiers, who could not produce weapons were excluded (Lowicki & Pillsbury, 2002; McKay & Mazurana, 2004). Additionally, funds for weapons were quickly exhausted (Lowicki & Pillsbury, 2002). Overall, this policy was inequitable.

Despite this, disarmament and demobilization was considered to be successful in some ways. According to Rugumamu and Gbla (2003), with the implementation process happening throughout various districts across Sierra Leone, confidence, understanding and trust were built within communities. In some districts, there were official public ceremonies where former combatants would take apart and destroy weapons, such as an AK-47, apologize, and swear an oath to peace.

The disarming process called for collaboration between local police and village elders. This in turn contributed to a stronger sense of security within a community. Additionally, a community could be declared 'weapons free', which gave it a certain status and helped to mobilize the community due to a sense of ownership (Kaldor & Vincent, 2006). Community members were more likely to report illicit weapons once they had been declared weapons free. Having a 'weapons free' status meant communities could choose projects for implementation, such as building a health centre, primary school or market centre.

Additionally, in terms of reestablishing some sense of authority and good governance, there was an emphasis on reviving the defunct local government system; thus, 96 paramount chiefs or regional chiefs returned to their chiefdoms, 50 district officials returned to their districts, and magistrate courts began operating again in most of the provinces (Rugumamu & Gbla, 2003). UNAMSIL played a critical role in facilitating this.

## The reintegration phase

The reintegration phase was critical to establishing and ensuring security and stability across the nation. At the same time, the nation of Sierra Leone was basically starting from scratch in the rebuilding process, as so much of the infrastructure had been destroyed through the 11-year war. There was a high priority on clean water distribution and electrical power delivery, along with ensuring that reintegration was working well, though without the latter the former would certainly be undermined.[9] That said, civil society members frequently reiterated that they wanted peace above all (Goins, 2015).

Relevant vocational training facilitated reintegration. Trained individuals could make a significant contribution to the community by putting their new skills to good use. Additionally, some former soldiers were given a small sum of money to start up a small business. This fostered good relationships and helped reintegration in some communities.[10] However, in others it fostered resentment, as those who did not participate in the atrocities of the war would have liked skills/vocational training. They felt the former soldiers were being privileged, almost rewarded for their part in destroying the country (Goins, 2015). That said, job training and placement is critical to good reintegration, particularly for youth and former child combatants. There was a scarcity of good opportunities for this population, and there continues to be. In 2001, 800,000 youth between the ages of 15 and 25 were unemployed, unpaid or underemployed. Currently, the youth unemployment rate (young people aged 15–35) is 60 per cent.[11]

Providing public information, community sensitization and reconciliation plans were all part of the strategy for the reintegration process (Goins, 2015). The Truth and Reconciliation Commission (TRC) facilitated this process, as did the Inter-Religious Council of Sierra Leone (IRCSL). The TRC addressed human rights violations and abuses and provided a forum for victims and offenders to tell their stories. The TRC hearings were open to the public and also broadcast within the districts in which they were held. There were other public radio broadcasts, public speeches made by travelling government figures, and outreaches into more rural villages and communities as well as populated cities and internally displaced persons' (IDP) camps through non-governmental agencies and civil society members (Goins, 2015).

The Special Court for Sierra Leone was established to try those guilty of war crimes in the Sierra Leone war. In April 2012, in The Hague, former president of Liberia Charles Taylor was found guilty of war crimes. The Revolutionary United Front leader, Foday Sankoh, was indicted for war crimes but never stood trial due to his death in 2003.

## Factors affecting reintegration and recovery

In the absence of a formal 'reintegration programme', reintegration still happened, both informally and through more focused efforts. However, practically speaking, there was not always a place to go. The destruction was so widespread that entire villages and communities no longer existed, particularly in the more rural areas of the country. By 2002, more than half of the population had been displaced.[12] Currently, poverty is heavily concentrated in rural areas and urban areas outside Freetown.[13] However, there was also the issue of the returnee having been part of the destruction process, in which case s/he would not necessarily be welcomed. New communities that formed in Freetown were a result of this factor, such as communities of former soldiers who chose to live together, communities of street children and young people, and communities within IDP camps.

Rape was prevalent during the war. Many females were sexually violated, in particular those who were recruited into fighting forces. (This was also the fate for males, though it was rarely talked about.)[14] In this case, they were used as sex slaves or bush wives. For the sake of their own protection, females would often attach themselves to one male as their husband and, ultimately, the father of their 'bush baby'. Rape being taboo, and given the shame associated with it, females felt they would be stigmatized and rejected by their families and communities because virginity is an important cultural value. The humiliation of rape is not just experienced by the victim but also by the victim's family, which carried significant implications for reintegration.

If 'bush babies' were involved, reintegration could be even more complicated. One girl said:

> My elder sister was captured by the rebels and taken to the bush. . . . The rebels impregnated her. My father, he would not allow her (the sister) into the house. Because he don't want that girl to give birth to a rebel child. So . . . he asks the girl out of the house. But I apologize on my sister's behalf, (but) my father gave me a big slap and my sister is in the streets right now.

> (Goins, 2015)

Former male soldiers had fears of being stigmatized too. Some reported that they 'would not get a good marriage' because it was assumed that having been a soldier, they had committed rape (Boyden, 2003). Others who had actually committed rape, though under severe duress, avoided those families and communities post-war, due to their own shame and fear of consequences (Goins, 2015).

## Conclusions

Post-conflict recovery for Sierra Leone was possible because of the international support that this country received (Kaldor & Vincent, 2006; Rugumamu & Gbla, 2003). Financial as well as capacity building support came through from various government and non-government agencies. However, it was not sustainable, and the government of Sierra Leone has been criticized for relying too much on '. . . external actors for post-war capacity building' (Rugumamu & Gbla, 2003, p. 33). Monies ended and programmes closed down with no good strategy for continuation of processes that had already begun. As Rugumamu and Gbla said,

'Successful post-war peace building and reconstruction hinges largely on the availability of funds, support and commitment to the realization of complete disarmament, demobilization and reintegration of former fighters' (2003, p. 33).[15]

Additionally, programme implementation was most often direct rather than through the Sierra Leone government. Thus, capacity building on a national level was hindered. That said, it was reported that civil society did not trust the government and preferred direct implementation (Kaldor & Vincent, 2006).

Youth engagement has been and will continue to be critical to long-term peace and recovery. Momoh from the Community Theatre Agency (CTA) noted that because of the new appointment of a youth minister, youth felt they were being listened to (Goins, 2015). Kaldor and Vincent (2006) recommended that various mechanisms for youth representation be created, so that youth will not be disenfranchised, as many complained they were before the war. That said, between 2009 and 2011, the UNDP managed a youth employment programme in Sierra Leone which increased income by 197 per cent.[16] This sounds like a huge increase; however, salaries are typically under US$2 a day for youth.

Also critical is consideration of building capacity for and supporting women and girls. They did not receive the attention nor services that males received post-war. There must be a greater effort made towards job creation for women (Kaldor & Vincent, 2006).

All in all, there is a long road ahead for Sierra Leone's post-war recovery. At the beginning of the war, Sierra Leone was ranked lowest on the United Nations Human Development Index. In 2012, it had moved up to 177 out of 187 countries. In 2014, it ranked at 183 out of 195 countries.[17] It is currently dealing with a health crisis that it is not equipped for, adding to the many systemic challenges this country faces in its post-war recovery.

In the next chapter, we will consider how children in particular were impacted by the 11-year war. Their stories bring to life some of the complexities to be considered around their recruitment, engagement and then recovery.

## Notes

1   Peters claims that two-thirds of the RUF were below 25 years old.
2   Available at: http://www.sierra-leone.org/lomeaccord.html [Accessed 15 April 2015].
3   Sierra Leonean civic groups played an important part in the peace negotiations. Perhaps the strongest player was the Inter-Religious Council of Sierra Leone (Adebajo, 2002). The IRCSL's members earned the confidence of both government and rebels during the 1996 Abidjan peace negotiations (Adebajo, 2002) and were thus a strong influence in the following years both in government and civil society.
4   Available at the following: http://reliefweb.int/report/guinea/uscr-country-report-sierra-leone-statistics-refugees-and-other-uprooted-people-jun; http://www.refworld.org/docid/40b459468.html [Accessed 5 August 2015].
5   Davies is a Sierra Leonean scholar Goins interviewed. Other interviewees confirmed this. (See also Appadurai, 1999; Baker & May, 2004; Bangura, 1997; Govier, 2006; Richards, 1996; Zack-Williams, 1999).
6   Available at: http://allafrica.com/stories/200410200357.html [Accessed 29 August 2014].

7   Of these, 6,316 were boys and 539 were girls who were registered through the DDRP. That said, the UNMIL (United Nations Mission in Liberia) reported that the number of girl soldiers who were disarmed and demobilized by UNMIL was also 539, which implies unreliability in either tracking or reporting disarmed children, particularly girls.

8   According to Professor Kenji Isezaki, who served as chief of the DDRP from May 2001 to January 2002.

9   The current power generation capacity is highly inadequate and unable to accommodate the country's needs. See: http://www.worldbank.org/en/country/sierraleone/overview [Accessed 28 September 2014].

10  This can be understood as part of a repentance process in the communal setting, which will be discussed further in another chapter.

11  See: http://www.worldbank.org/en/country/sierraleone/overview [Accessed 28 September 2014].

12  Available at: http://web.undp.org/evaluation/documents/thematic/conflict/sierraleone.pdf [Accessed 5 August 2015].

13  See: http://www.worldbank.org/en/country/sierraleone/overview [Accessed 28 September 2014].

14  Due to the fear of being stigmatized as a homosexual, males who had been raped rarely spoke of it. See: http://www.hrw.org/reports/2003/sierraleone/sierleon0103.pdf.

15  Complete report available at: http://www.lencd.org/files/casestory/Studies_in_reconstruction_and_capacity_building_in_post-conflict_countries_in_Africa:_some_lessons_of_experience_from_Sierra_Leone/14-Post_Conflict_Study_Report_on_Sierra_Leone.pdf.

16  See Sierra Leone Youth Report/Youth Development (2012). Available in pdf: http://www.sl.undp.org/content/dam/sierraleone/docs/projectdocuments/povreduction/sl_status_ofthe_youth_report2012FINAL.pdf [Accessed 28 September 2014].

17  See: http://www.worldbank.org/en/country/sierraleone/overview [Accessed 28 September 2014]. See the most current report available at: http://hdr.undp.org/en/countries [Accessed 14 March 2015].

## References

Abdullah, I. (1997) Bush path to destruction: The origin and character of the Revolutionary United Front (RUF/SL). *Africa Development,* 22(3/4): 45–76.

Abdullah, I., Muana, P. (1998) The Revolutionary United Front of Sierra Leone: A revolt of the Lumpen-proletariat. In C. Clapham (Ed.), *African guerrillas* (pp. 173–193). Oxford: James Currey Ltd.

Abraham, A. (2001) Dancing with the chameleon: Sierra Leone and the elusive quest for peace. *Journal of Contemporary African Studies,* 19(2): 206–228.

Adebajo, A. (2002) *Building peace in West Africa: Liberia, Sierra Leone, and Guinea Bissau.* Boulder, CO: Lynne Rienner.

Appadurai, A. (1999) Dead certainty: Ethnic violence in the era of globalization. In B. Meyer, P. Geschiere (Eds.), *Globalization and identity: Dialectics of flow and closure* (pp. 305–324). Oxford: Blackwell Publishers.

Baker, B., May, R. (2004) Reconstructing Sierra Leone. *Commonwealth & Comparative Politics,* 42(1): 35–60.

Baksh-Soodeen, R., Etchart, L. (2001) *Women and men in partnership for post-conflict reconstruction.* London: Commonwealth Secretariat.

Bangura, Y. (1997) Understanding the political and cultural dynamics of the Sierra Leonean war: A critique of Paul Richard's 'Fighting for the Rain Forest'. *Africa Development,* 22(3 & 4): 117–148.

Boyden, J. (2003) The moral development of child soldiers: what do adults have to fear? *Peace and Conflict: Journal of Peace Psychology,* 9(4): 343–362.

Campbell, G. (2002) *Blood diamonds: Tracing the deadly path of the world's most precious stones.* Cambridge, MA: Westview Press Books.

Chege, M. (2002) The state that came back from the dead. *The Washington Quarterly,* 25(3): 147–160.

CSUCS (Coalition to Stop the Use of Child Soldiers) (2003) *Guide to the optional protocol on the involvement of children in armed conflict.* New York: UNICEF.

CSUCS (Coalition to Stop the Use of Child Soldiers) (2004) *Child soldiers global report 2004; 10 January 2005.* New York: UNICEF.

Davies, V. (2002) *War, poverty and growth in Africa: Lessons in Sierra Leone.* Paper presented at the Conference on Understanding Poverty and Growth in Africa, Oxford University.

Forna, A. (2002) *The devil that danced on the water: A daughter's memoir of her father, her family, her country and a continent.* London: HarperCollins Publishers.

Gberie, L. (2004) Sierra Leone's TRC report: Preliminary comments. *Concord Times.* Freetown: Concord Times.

Gbla, O. (2003) Conflict and post-war trauma among child soldiers in Liberia and Sierra Leone. In A. Sesay (Ed.), *Civil wars, child soldiers and post conflict peace building in West Africa* (pp. 167–194). Ibadan, Nigeria: Nigerian College Press Publishers.

Glover, R. D. (1999) Small minds and big hearts: Prospects for sustainable peace in Sierra Leone. *The Richardson Institute papers* No. 1999/1.40. Lancaster: Lancaster University.

Goins, S. (2015) *Forgiveness and reintegration: How the transformative process of forgiveness impacts child soldier reintegration* (provisional title). Oxford,: Regnum Books.

Govier, T. (2006) *Taking wrongs seriously: Acknowledgment, reconciliation, and the politics of sustainable peace.* Amherst, NY: Humanity Books.

Hirsch, J. L. (2001) *Sierra Leone: Diamonds and the struggle for democracy.* London: Lynne Rienner Publishers.

HRW (Human Rights Watch) (1999) *World Report: Sierra Leone.* Available at: http://www.hrw.org/legacy/wr2k/Africa-09.htm [Accessed 5 August 2015].

ICG (International Crisis Group) (2001) *Sierra Leone: Managing uncertainty in Africa Report No. 35.* Brussels: International Crisis Group.

Jackson, M. (2004) *In Sierra Leone.* Durham, NC: Duke University Press.

Kaldor, M., Vincent, J. (2006) *Evaluation of UNDP assistance to conflict-affected countries: Case study Sierra Leone.* United Nations Development Programme. Available at: http://web.undp.org/evaluation/documents/thematic/conflict/SierraLeone.pdf [Accessed 21 September 2014].

Kandeh, J. D. (2002) Subaltern terror in Sierra Leone. In A. Zack-Williams, D. Frost, A. Thomson (Eds.), *Africa in crisis: New challenges and possibilities* (pp. 179–195). London: Pluto Press.

Kandeh, J. D. (2003) Sierra Leone's post-conflict elections of 2002. *The Journal of Modern African Studies,* 41(2): 189–216.

Keen, D. (2005) *The best of enemies: Conflict and collusion in Sierra Leone.* Oxford: James Currey Ltd.

Lowicki, J., Pillsbury, A. A. (2002) *Precious resources: Adolescents in the reconstruction of Sierra Leone.* New York: Women's Commission for Refugee Women and Children.

Lyon, J. A. (2004) Gender-based violence and biblical equality: Case studies in Sierra Leone. *Priscilla Papers,* 18: 3–6.

Mawson, A., Dodd, R., Hilary, J. (2000) *War brought us here.* London: Save the Children.

Mazurana, D., Carlson, K. (2004) *From combat to community: Women and girls of Sierra Leone.* Available at: www.huntalternativesfund.org and www.womenwagingpeace.net [Accessed 7 February 2006].

McKay, S., Mazurana, D. (2004) *Where are the girls? Girls in fighting forces in Northern Uganda, Sierra Leone and Mozambique: Their lives during and after war.* Montreal: International Centre for Human Rights and Democratic Development.

Noyes, F. (2003) Preventive diplomacy in Sierra Leone. In H. Solomon (Ed.), *Towards sustainable peace: The theory and practice of preventive diplomacy in Africa* (pp. 44–101). Pretoria: Africa Institute of South Africa.

Olonisakin, F. (2000) *Engaging Sierra Leone. CDD strategy planning series 2000.* London: Centre for Democracy and Development.

Peters, K. (2006) *Footpaths to reintegration: Armed conflict, youth and the rural crisis in Sierra Leone.* Wageningen, Holland: Wageningen University.

Peters, K., Richards, P. (1998) Fighting with open eyes: Young combatants talking about war in Sierra Leone. In P.C.P. Bracken (Ed.), *Rethinking the trauma of war* (pp. 76–111). London: Free Association Books.

Physicians for Human Rights (PHR) (2003) *War-related sexual violence in Sierra Leone.* Washington, DC: UNAMSIL & PHR.

Reno, W. (1995) *Corruption and state politics in Sierra Leone.* Cambridge: Cambridge University Press.

Revolutionary United Front (RUF) (1995) *Footpaths to democracy toward a new Sierra Leone.* Available at: http://fas.org/irp/world/para/docs/footpaths.htm [Accessed 5 August 2015].

Richards, P. (1996) *Fighting for the rain forest.* London: Villiers Publications.

Rosen, D. M. (2005) *Armies of the young: Child soldiers in war and terrorism.* New Brunswick, NJ: Rutgers University Press.

Rugumamu, S., Gbla, O. (2003) *Studies in reconstruction and capacity building in post-conflict countries in Africa: Some lessons of experience from Sierra Leone. The African Capacity Building Foundation.* Harare, Zimbabwe: The African Capacity Building Foundation.

Sesay, O. F. (2004) Stopping circles of impunity? *Peep! Magazine,* 3: 3, 8. Freetown.

Shepler, S. (2005) *Conflicted childhoods: Fighting over child soldiers in Sierra Leone.* Unpublished Doctor of Philosophy, University of California at Berkeley, Berkeley.

TRC (2004) *Truth and Reconciliation Commission report.* Accra: International Human Rights Law Group.

United Nations (1999) *Disarmament, demobilisation, and reintegration of ex-combatants in a peacekeeping environment: Principles and guidelines.* 112: Department of Peacekeeping Operations. Available at: www.somali-jna.org [Accessed 2 May 2015].

Weissman, V. W. (2003) Sierra Leone: Peace at any price. In F. Weissman (Ed.), *In the shadow of 'just' wars* (pp. 43–65). London: Hurst & Company.

Williamson, J., Cripe, L. (2002) *Assessment of DCOF-supported child demobilization and reintegration activities in Sierra Leone.* Washington, DC: US Agency for International Development.

World Bank (2002) *Sierra Leone: Disarmament, demobilisation and reintegration (DDR). Good practice info brief.* Africa Region: World Bank.

Zack-Williams, A. B. (1999) Sierra Leone: The political economy of civil war, 1991–98. *Third World Quarterly,* 20(1): 143–162.

Zack-Williams, A. B. (2001) Child soldiers in the civil war in Sierra Leone. *Review of African Political Economy,* 87: 73–82.

# Part 2

# Survivors' stories

# Chapter 5

# Child soldiers' stories
## Killing was the order of the day

'*Killing was the order of the day.*' This is what Sorie[1] told one of us (Stephanie Goins), as he recounted what he had witnessed prior to his abduction, and what he experienced during his time with the Revolutionary United Front (RUF). His story was typical.

Sorie was living in Freetown in January 1999 when the infamous RUF invasion took place. He had relocated from a northern province in order to continue his secondary education, already interrupted several times due to the war. During that invasion, Sorie was abducted. When the RUF learnt that Sorie was a pastor's son, 'they were very happy (because) they needed someone to pray for them in the bush' (Goins, 2015).[2] With Sorie being Christian, his 'purity' was presumed. This additional feature made Sorie a desirable recruit, promising protection from evil, harmful spirits and failure in battle.

Sorie's primary role was as the group's pastor. His purity should be protected or the group's success would be put at risk. In reality, what it meant was that Sorie would not be forced to kill anyone. The day Sorie was abducted 'was the saddest day' of his life.

> I was going to a destination where I knew nobody and where killing was the order of the day. I did not even think of seeing my brothers, sisters, friends and the rest of my family again. It was a time of bitter crying with a bag of rice on my head as we were going to the bush. It was after 75 miles walking on my legs before we could rest.

Sorie's indoctrination into the RUF was through a combination of training, violence and violations. For three weeks, he endured 'serious beatings on his back'. He was forced to commit acts that were a serious violation of his conscience. Sorie, who began his RUF life as a victim, would soon become a perpetrator (Goins, 2015).

While his 'purity' was to be protected, the rebels were more determined to ensure his loyalty.

> It was on the 23rd February 1999 that I went through the initiation process with the rebels and one of them I will never forget in my life time. It was a 12-year-old girl that I was forced to rape. It was not an easy task for me. I refused to do that but they

*threatened to kill me with a gunshot on the ground under my feet. . . . They forced me to the point that I found no option. The girl did cry and I cried with her too because she was too small, and the worst thing they did was that I would take an hour complete.*

*On that same day, I was forced again to rape an old woman who was even older than my mother. . . . Well, it's too hard to explain. At times when I remembered that scene, I cried seriously and up to now I have never gone to the area where it happened. Being afraid that they will point fingers on me and because of that I still hold these people in my mind.*

It was three years later when Sorie relayed his story. He had never told anyone. The initiation had silenced him, instilling a deep sense of shame and reinforcing the fear already in him (Goins, 2015).

Sorie was not only the pastor but also the cook.

*One day the cooking items were not enough so that when I cooked, it was not all that sweet. They were very angry with me and punished me. The punishment was to burn down a village of 35 houses to ash. They gave me a gallon of petrol and a box of matches.*

Obviously, what it means to 'protect purity' is relative to the interpreter.

As their pastor, Sorie's responsibility was to prepare sermons. His sermons did not present a conflict to this mix of Muslims, Christians and animists. He prayed for encouragement and their success as they went into battle. However, on one occasion, Sorie did not pray 'well enough' and was required to participate in battle. During this battle, he was separated from the group for several days. He did not try to escape because he had a young boy with him. If discovered, he knew they would be killed or severely punished.

However, there soon came another opportunity. Sorie escaped with a small amount of money, which covered his travel on the back of a lorry. He was excited beyond words to be escaping and, at the same time, frightened beyond words that he would be caught.

Sorie arrived in Freetown without resources. Because he had no weapon, he could not apply for the Disarmament, Demobilization, and Reintegration programme. Returning to the province where his family lived would have been dangerous and impractical, so he lived with a relative. He was grateful, but 'not happy' because she did not like him.

When Sorie eventually saw his family, there was little mention of his time with the RUF except to ask, 'Why are you fat?'. He explained that he was the cook, which satisfied them. Questions about killing, rape, arson, looting, amputating, or any offences that were commonly associated with the RUF never came up in conversation.[3]

Several months later, he moved into a compound with other former child soldiers. He felt welcomed and understood (Goins, 2015). He became involved in his church youth group and eventually became its president. He said, 'I am blessed with the things of God. In my church everybody loves me. . . . And I see myself leading wherever I find myself.'

Being now free for more than a year and having had time to consider what he had done, Sorie felt deep guilt. While he would never have committed these offences had he not been abducted, the fact is that he did.[4] The two offences that weighed heaviest on him were the rapes. He wanted to be forgiven, to have the shame lifted from him, not to be excluded from the community, and to make things right.[5]

Sorie would never return to the village where he raped the elderly woman. The shame around this event was nearly unbearable. However, having confessed to his pastor about the 12-year-old girl, Sorie (along with his pastor) returned to her community. Sorie asked the girl and her family, who had witnessed the rape, for forgiveness. By this time, Sorie had received sponsorship to attend Fourah Bay College in Freetown. The family saw that Sorie would have a bright future and believed he would be a good marriage partner for their daughter, a kind of restitution for the violation. Sorie said,

> Because of that (raping a virgin) the custom says that I should marry the girl. To satisfy them, I answered yes and the girl is waiting for me to marry her one day after (I finish) school. That I will not do (marry her) and (they) will curse me. . . . The mistake I did was to go and ask for forgiveness.

Sorie said he is praying 'for a way of escape'. He fears being cursed for not following through with the marriage. Curses '. . . are considered to be one among the four major causes of death' (Finnegan, 1964, p. 24). Though not his first choice, if need be, he would even leave his beloved country.

Sorie's story is representative of many children recruited into the various armed groups fighting during the 11-year civil war. His life was dramatically disrupted, though for a relatively short period of time in comparison to some other recruited children. Some were involved in the war for years; some would have been recruited as children but demobilized as adults.

In many ways, Sorie was fortunate. He was never forced to kill or maim. His offences were carried out against people he did not know. He had a place to go after his escape. He could actually begin to rebuild his life, with the help and support of others who welcomed him, understood him and provided for him. As Stephanie's fieldwork revealed, other former child soldiers were not so fortunate. What now follows in this chapter are stories of former child soldiers whose lives, experiences and future hopes are both similar and different to those of Sorie. However, before beginning with these stories, we will briefly discuss the approach taken in collecting data through narratives, interviews, focus groups and repertory grid technique.

## Research method

### Participants

The participants came from various parts of the country and were living in Freetown at the time of the study. The sample population was made up of adults and children from different ethnic groups who practised various religions. Both combatants and ex-combatants, as well as people with various positions in civil society, were part of the study. Expatriates, primarily those working with international non-governmental organizations (INGOs) in or around Freetown, provided data. Most interviewees were Sierra Leonean. Where interviews were conducted outside of Sierra Leone, those interviewees had lived in various parts of the country. Some girls and women were from the Cline Town IDP (internally displaced persons) camp located in Freetown. Some of those girls and women had children. Most were at least slightly illiterate.

The total sample size, including those who provided written discourse or repertory grids, totalled 322. Of those, there were 135 males, 129 under 18 years old. There were 187 females, 154 under 18 years old. Overall, the ages ranged from 10 to 30 years old; and of those, 201 were between the ages of 12 to 15 years.

### Narratives

The written material, including self-characterizations and narratives, was collected from two segments of the population: children from three different schools and residents of the Cline Town IDP camp. Over the three different sessions, individuals who produced narratives were first asked to provide a self-characterization in which they would write three things about themselves that the researcher would not know. This could be written in the first person or the third person; however, if the latter, it would be from an individual who knows them 'intimately and sympathetically'. In the second session, these same individuals were asked the following question: 'Tell me a story about the war that you can easily forgive and tell me why you can easily forgive it.' In the third session, the question to answer was as follows: 'Tell me a story about the war that you cannot easily forgive and tell me why you cannot easily forgive it.'

Due to support from the supervisor for the Ministry of Education, access was gained to two primary schools and one secondary school. Work with the IDP camp residents was enabled through Action for People in Conflict (AfPiC), who had a programme operating in the IDP camp but nothing geared towards meeting the psychosocial needs of the female attendees.

### Interviews

Sixteen interviews were conducted by Stephanie during the time of her fieldwork in Sierra Leone and 15 conducted since. Of the interviewees who provided data in Sierra Leone, 13 were nationals and 3 were expatriates who lived and worked in Sierra Leone. Data from interviews conducted outside Sierra Leone came from 14 nationals who had either moved away from Sierra Leone permanently or were living in England for a period of time before returning to Sierra Leone. One remaining expatriate was interviewed outside Sierra Leone but had lived and worked in Sierra Leone. The majority of interviewees had experienced the war first-hand.

Interviews were face-to-face and lasted from 20 minutes to several hours. Some people were interviewed several times. There was a list of questions, which was generally followed, though at times asking these specific questions was not necessary or possible, as the interviewee was moving from topic to topic. The interviewee usually received a list of questions prior to the interview in order to prepare him or her and make best use of our time.[6]

## Focus groups

Focus group discussions were conducted in two classes at a primary school (varying between 35 and 45 students) and three sessions at the IDP camp (the first with approximately 25 females, the second with approximately 15, and the third with 10).

For each focus group, the topic of forgiveness was introduced as the focal point of discussion. The group was guided towards the questions of interest. Overall, group members seemed open and eager to speak. The children were generally polite and waited for one another to finish before speaking out. Their discussions generally lasted 45 minutes. The focus groups with the IDP residents lasted anywhere from 1 hour 15 minutes to 1 hour 45 minutes. The participants were more spontaneous than the children. The IDP discussions were recorded and also translated.

For the first two meetings, the IDP residents related stories of their experiences in the war. The same general format was used as with the narratives that had been requested from the children. The third focus group meeting with the IDP residents explored a phrase that had been repeated in casual conversations and in the children's narratives: I forgive but I'll never forget. There were two focus group discussions conducted with the children in their classrooms. The number of participants varied from 35 to 45. Both group discussions opened with the same question, with the discussion being guided in order to cover other topics.[7]

## Repertory grids

Thirty-four grids were collected from three groups. Group 1 had 12 participants, half of whom had been combatants (two males and four females). Group 2 had 10 participants, all female former combatants. Group 3 had 12 participants, five male and three female former combatants. Groups 1 and 3 were students from the secondary school. Group 2 participants were IDP camp residents.

Repertory grid technique (Fransella, Bell & Bannister, 2004) is the principal assessment method derived from Kelly's (1955) personal construct theory (see Chapter 2), and was employed to investigate the construing of the research participants, particularly in relation to how they saw themselves. The flexibility of this technique, and its focus on the individuals' view of the world in their own terms rather than in terms of the investigator's constructs, makes it well suited to research in different cultural settings, and it had been previously used in studies in Africa (Orley, 1976; Veale, 2003), including one on former child soldiers.

The technique involves eliciting from the individuals a set of elements of their experience (generally other people and aspects of the self) and then sorting these in terms of a set of bipolar constructs, which are generally elicited from the individuals by asking them to compare and contrast the elements. This procedure was modified somewhat in the current study in view of feedback from piloting of the grid and because conditions were such that only group administration of the grid was possible. The principal modification was that the constructs were supplied to, rather than elicited from, the participants, but ensuring their relevance by deriving them from descriptors that were used repeatedly in participants' interviews, narratives and focus groups. The constructs used with Group 1 were *forgiving – takes revenge, deserves to be forgiven – doesn't deserve forgiveness, thankful – ungrateful, afraid – fearless,*[8] *sad – happy, forced – willing, suffers – enjoys, responsible – not responsible,*[9] *kind – bad* and *powerful – weak.*[10] In Groups 2 and 3, *forced – willing* was replaced by *guilty – not guilty*. The elements were *me before the war, me now, me during the war, me 10 years from now, how I should be, how I would like to be, a good friend, a victim, my commanding officer,* and *my guardian* or *someone who sympathizes with me*. Since it transpired that *how I should be* and *how I would like to be* were indistinguishable by participants in Group 1, the latter element was replaced by *how a family member sees me* in Group 2 and by *a volunteer* (someone who was not abducted) in Group 3. During the piloting of the grid, participants were asked to rate all of the elements on all of the constructs, using a 7-point scale. However, since they experienced difficulties in using this scale, in the main study rating was replaced by Kelly's original procedure of asking participants to allocate each element to one or the other pole of each construct.

Various software packages were used to derive measures from the grid.[11] The HICLAS package (deBoeck, 1986) provided a measure of the degree of elaboration of *me during the war*, essentially indicating the extent to which constructs could be applied to this element. The GRIDCOR package (Feixas and Cornejo, 2002) allowed derivation of measures of distance between (i.e., dissimilarity in construing of) pairs of elements and pairs of constructs; as well as intensity, the sum of squares of correlations between constructs, and the percentage of variance accounted for by the first axis of correspondence analysis of the grid, both of these latter measures providing an indication of the tightness of, or lack of differentiation in, the individual's construing. The Idiogrid package (Grice, 2002) was used to calculate correlations between constructs and to conduct a principal components analysis, which essentially identifies the major dimensions in the grid and provides a plot of the elements and constructs along these dimensions. The proximity of elements and constructs in the plot is assumed to reflect their psychological proximity. Finally, the GRIDSTAT package (Bell, 2009) was used to derive a measure of conflict, or logical inconsistency, in construing.

## More stories of former child soldiers

We shall now present further stories elicited by the narratives and focus groups.

### The longing for education

Most former child soldiers were enrolled in school before the war began. There was a high value placed on education, though admittedly schools were run-down and without resources, while teachers were often ill equipped and some even apathetic. The longing to go to school was expressed repeatedly in children's narratives, focus groups, and interviews. Children talked about their favourite subjects, sports, how clever they were, and how hard they worked in school. When primary education was completed, they were sent to another province to continue with secondary education. This was the expected way of life for urban children, and the desired way of life for rural children.

Many children experienced disrupted education because of the movement of the war. OK,[12] a 14-year-old boy, was captured by the RUF after they killed his father, mother and sister. He managed to escape and was being cared for by his brother at the time of his interview. He said he was forced to beg, as were many children. He was also forced to sit in a classroom with children four to five years younger than him, and considerably smaller, which for some boys was particularly humiliating.[13]

### Circumstantial recruitment

Many children were vulnerable to recruitment due to their being gathered in one place, such as a school. This was the case for Momoh.[14] He lived in a province and was attending a secondary school some distance from his village when the RUF invaded. Some of his friends were abducted. Momoh was the family member designated to join the village civil defence force (CDF), which meant he would sometimes be fighting against his schoolmates. This was all too often the case for children involved in war. Momoh, like most children, did not want to be involved in war but had no choice.

Other children chose to, though we use the word 'chose' loosely here. OD,[15] an 18-year-old former child soldier, was abducted at 14 years old. When he managed to escape, he joined a CDF in retaliation. Clearly his time as a soldier caused internal conflict, as he wrote the following: '*I am appealing to everybody that know that I have done bad to him, let he/she forgive me.*'

## Roles and functions

Once children had been recruited into an armed group, they filled various roles and functions, including typical 'chores' done at home. Both boys and girls were responsible for doing things such as fetching water, scrounging for food, cooking, or doing laundry. *'The RUF captured me, take me as a dish man,'* said a 15-year-old boy.[16] Both boys and girls were responsible for these duties (Goins, 2015).

## A fictive community life

Typically, armed groups lived in camps that were set apart from other villages. This created a fictive community, where purportedly there were familial relationships. Male commanders were 'fathers'; Mammy Queens[17] were 'mothers' and keepers of the children; and the children were siblings. Again purportedly, there was to be sexual abstinence between males and females, unless the female's role was as a 'bush wife' (Gbla, 2003). However, female former child soldiers provided much more evidence of sexual violations that occurred, definitely outside the definition of a 'sibling' relationship (Goins, 2015).

Within this community, as Sorie's story illustrated, there may have been someone to conduct a religious or spiritual service of some kind, prayer or preaching. There would be ceremonies where evil spirits were warded off. Recruits worshipped according to their religious preference. Peters and Richards (1998) said children were obligated to pray.

Perhaps this alludes to a more normalized picture of children and wartime experiences. For some children who were abducted at a very young age, that may have been their experience. One boy was abducted at six years old.[18] He was awaiting reunification with his family, after having been with the RUF for eight years. He had little memory of them and no recollection of where he was from. The armed group had become his family. Though life was anything but 'normal', it was what he had known; it was his 'normal'.

Many children talked about seeing family members killed, leaving them extremely vulnerable and most often without any resources, as was expressed by this 17-year-old male former soldier:

> *I we not forgive the rebel kill my father because it is my father only who is going to take care of me, my plans [for] tomorrow. He was the only one that can take care of me and my young sister and elder brother. Also my mother the rebel kill her. They burn our house and burn grandfather in the house. He likes me and also I like him so much. My father is the only one who is going to take care of me about my school problems and take care of my clothes . . . now I did not have anybody to take care of me like my father. . . . Can you imagine all the things my father does for me. How can I forgive these peoples like that. They kill my father and burn my grandfather who [liked] me very much. [With] all the things that have happened to me, how can I feel happy [when] they kill my father and my grandfather.[19]*

### Experiences of violence

For many female former child soldiers who were living in the Cline Town IDP camp, a sense of family might have reluctantly been created but with very violent beginnings. Stephanie's field data confirmed that a girl's introduction to the armed group often, though not always, came through sexual violence (Goins, 2015). Following that, girls were nearly always given to commanders as wives or girlfriends, or used as sexual slaves:

> The rebels . . . captured me . . . alongside my mother and I was raped. So, the one that raped me was the boss of the rebels. . . . (T)hree of them were fighting for me. They said they want me to be their wife. So I was impregnated by the boss of the rebels. He finally succeeded in getting me.[20]

Females at the IDP camp all had similar stories of sexual assault. If possible, they attached themselves to one rebel in order to be protected from gang rape or other kinds of harm. One IDP resident was in her mid-teens when her parents were killed and she was raped. She said her best alternative was 'to join them because of the fearness in me'.[21] Several girls wrote about being abducted or raped, or losing one or both parents, as exemplified below:

> When the rebel took me to the bush on that day, I am in my house and all my family. My mother is cooking. . . . Then we heard gun sound. . . . The rebel came and push the door, and [they were] shooting. I was behind the door . . . and (the rebel) found me and take me . . . to the bush and I begin to shout. Then he told me to naked myself and I say to them, please sir forgive me sir (according to her and in other words, 'please leave me alone'), and they left me [so I could] come home.[22]

Unfortunately, her experience did not end here, as she was later abducted and raped.

Contrary to Sorie's overall experience, the violence that children experienced could only be described as horrific. FM, at the time around 13 years old, described how she and her mother were captured by the RUF. Her mother, six months pregnant, was sent to look for food and tried to escape but was recaptured.

> The rebels were having a young boy who was . . . called a commando and he was in charge of tearing peoples' stomachs to see what was inside. He decided that they should tear my mother's stomach so they see what's inside there because she (my mother) will not be able to travel with them. . . . That boy took the knife and said, 'Because we do not have any . . . meat for the sauce, we should tear this stomach and find out what is inside there for the sauce.' He took the knife and did the action and find a small, premature baby having only a foot inside my mother's belly. After my mother was killed by them, they (the rebels) asked me, 'Why are you so sad? If you

*are sad you will follow your mother, so it will be better for you to be happy.' I decided, 'I'm not sad, I'm happy.' So they said, 'If you're happy, come and join us in eating.'*[23]

This was, unfortunately, a typical story. Children were powerless, and females usually more so because of the additional sexual violence perpetrated upon them. That said, boys were also subjected to sexual violence, particularly as an initiation tactic.

As was Sorie's experience, children were forced to burn houses or villages, sometimes those belonging to family or community members. A 10-year-old male former soldier who was living in a province at the time said the following:

> *He (a rebel boy and former friend of this child) say . . . I must obey him because he is the master. . . . (H)e said, let me burn the house of my father. I said no, I will not do that, and he said, if I don't do that he will kill me and he give me the petrol and the gun and I threw the petrol in front of the parlour and I shoot. The fire began to blaze that time everything is inside the house, everything burn . . .*[24]

The RUF intentionally recruited children in order to '. . . break down the community fabric by letting the young decide over the life and death of adults' (Boyden, 2003, p. 346). Children were used to target chiefs, traditional leaders such as imams or priests, prosperous farmers and traders (Abraham, 2001, p. 207). Children killed family or villagers, burned houses or villages, and raped, activities that have been documented in various sources (Gbla, 2003; Govier, 2006; HRW, 2001; Zack-Williams, 2001), as well as Stephanie's field data.

One 15-year-old male former soldier wrote, *'On the way to the battle we met one old grandmother and [the rebel] said to me let me shoot the grandmother. That is my grandmother and I cry.'*[25] Another 10-year-old child wrote, *'(The rebels take) my brother and give him gun and give him blood to drink but he did not drink it. And they command him to kill his uncle and father . . .'* Yet another boy, abducted at nine years old, wrote, *'I broke a woman's leg but not with my heart . . .'*[26] Oftentimes children, having killed family or community members, found it particularly difficult to reintegrate once the war ended.

### Drugs, alcohol and disfigurements

Drugs were frequently part of the wartime experience, as soldiers had ready access to drugs and alcohol (Zack-Williams, 2001). In fact, most interviewees and many children from SG's data pool assumed that if a child was fighting, s/he was concurrently using drugs. Marijuana was freely available, as were other drug and substance mixtures such as gunpowder and cocaine, making what is called 'brown-brown'. According to interviewees, these were used before and during fighting. Lowicki and Pillsbury (2002, p. 29) reported one adolescent saying, 'I became mad if I took too many drugs. I didn't care about things when I took drugs.' Substance dependency became an issue and purportedly, drug use increased once the war ended (Bennett, 2002; Goins, 2015; Lowicki & Pillsbury, 2002).

While drugs were often used for initiation and indoctrination tactics, so was disfigurement. RUF recruits were often tattooed with 'RUF' on their chests, predominantly males but also females. This would ensure their being killed by opposing forces (Govier, 2006). One 15-year-old girl who had been abducted showed Stephanie the initials 'RUF' carved into her chest. Her affect showed her to be traumatized.[27] In her narrative, she talked about being haunted by a wicked spirit that tried to get her to do things against her will. In summary, the establishment of a fictive family,[28] violence, the use of drugs and disfigurements are all practices purposed to secure the child's loyalty and obedience.

### Rehabilitation and reintegration challenges

Having experienced all this and more, once the war ended, integration into community life for former child soldiers was riddled with complexities. For some children such as this 18-year-old male,[29] the DDR programme helped immensely. Though he was abducted and obviously burdened by his involvement in the war, what he called 'guidance counselling' made him determined to put the past behind him and not fight again.

If a former child soldier had reasonable alternatives once the war ended, successful reintegration and rehabilitation were much more likely. It took much work on the part of all – the child who may have aged into adulthood, the receiving family/community, the village elders and chiefs, the agencies working with the child and family/community, and other civil society members. However, post-war recovery is complicated at best; a civil war is particularly complex in that the very fabric of society, along with its basic infrastructure, is often destroyed.

To help illustrate one of the complexities, Bishop Biguzzi, head of the Roman Catholic Diocese of Makini, said the following:

> One of the worst things from the war is the systematic undermining of the traditional culture. Respect for pregnant women and elders has totally disappeared. In the past, you wouldn't even speak to a senior. Now, child soldiers are cutting off the noses of village elders, forcing chiefs to undress in public. This is the worst form of humiliation for a Sierra Leonean.
> (Voeten, 2000, p. 202)

Children were also appalled by the role reversal.

*One boy came, a very small boy, [and] take a stick and hit my father [who] fell down, and [the boy] gave [my father] a load to carry. We carried it for 3 miles away. (On the way) [my father] met his smaller sister. His sister started crying [and said] take the load from my father's head. . . . The thing that I cannot forget [about] this story: Imagine that a small boy take a stick and hit my father with it.*[30]

Certainly both rehabilitation and reintegration are significantly challenged with the breakdown of cultural norms and traditions, the loss of respect for elders and religious leaders, the empowerment of child soldiers, and the resultant fears associated with them. Additionally, once the war ended, many former child soldiers who were used to looting, having food and money, and using violence to get what they wanted found it difficult to adjust to a different sort of life.

Several non-governmental organizations in Sierra Leone worked with both former child soldiers and their awaiting families and communities to address some of these complexities. Programmes within centres such as the Family Home Movement (FHM) and the Nehemiah Rehabilitation Project (NRP) were structured so as to incorporate traditional values and family/community life, love and concern for the child. Former child soldiers who went through the programme had ample opportunities for informal counselling, vocational skills training, spiritual pursuits, recreational activities, and so on. Father Chema Caballero[31] directed the FHM programme. He said the following:

*We were not just covering an office, we were sharing our life and home with them. This gave the children a sense of belonging in a family and provided them with some people they could trust. They could . . . open up and talk with the people in charge of the programme and share their experiences. . . . Children needed time and a person to trust, to open up and share their experiences, what they had gone through.*

Father Chema said this was 'a magic moment . . . the beginning of rehabilitation', which came when others were not around:

*The story of their fears and sufferings, the hunger, the cold, the beatings, the hate. What kept them alive during all this time: the desire to see his/her mother, his/her relatives, the desire of revenge, to kill the person who killed his/her father, who burnt down the family house, to get the chance to kill the person that kidnapped him/her, or sometimes the wish to go back to school . . .*

The family-like structure and the presence of caring adults helped prepare former child soldiers for reintegration. Additionally, both Father Chema and Richard Cole,[32] the cofounder and director of the NRP, would arrange meetings between former child soldiers in their programmes and the receiving communities. The NRP went a step further, in that programme participants learnt vocational skills that were of practical use to them and to the receiving communities. In one community, they built a school; in another community, they built a clinic.

Certainly post-war life was simpler for males than females. Many female former child soldiers had experienced sexual violence, and often had children, or 'bush babies'. Nearly every interviewee who spoke of these females and their children said they would suffer stigmatization and likely be shunned by their communities, though obviously their plights were not their own choosing.

IDP camp residents expressed their desire to be married and have families, but they felt that being victims of rape left them with little hope of a normal life.[33] This was even more the case for females who suffered from vaginal fistula as a result of rape. At that time, they could not envision ever returning to their communities. Additionally, females were less likely to receive vocational training, which left them with few alternatives to make a living.

## Repertory grid results

### Group data

Contrary to our predictions, there was no difference between the former combatants and the noncombatants in the degree of elaboration of the self during the war[34] (Goins, Winter, Sundin, Patient & Aslan, 2012). Even more surprisingly, the former combatants saw themselves now and during the war as more similar to how they should be than did the noncombatants.[35] Changes in the distance between the self at different time points and 'how I should be' in the two groups are shown in Figure 5.1. A mixed between-within subjects analysis of variance carried out on these scores indicated a significant interaction between combatant status and time[36] and significant main effects for combatant status[37] and time.[38] As further indicated by pairwise comparisons, all participants construed themselves during the war as less similar to how they should be than themselves before the war, but the difference was less marked in the former combatants.[39] The former combatants also viewed themselves now as even closer to how they should be than themselves before the war,[40] but this difference was not significant in the noncombatants. All participants anticipated that over the next 10 years they would become closer to how they should be,[41] and both viewed their future self as significantly closer to how they should be than was their pre-war self, but this difference was much greater in the former combatants.[42]

Other differences between the groups were that the former combatants had somewhat tighter construct systems, as indicated by the percentage of variance accounted for by the first axis from correspondence analysis of their grids,[43] and construed forgiveness rather more favourably, associating it with kindness and being thankful.[44] The female former combatants in the displacement camp had construct systems that were particularly tight, as indicated by the intensity measure, and free of conflict, compared to other female former combatants,[45] as well as more elaborated construing of the self during the war.[46]

In summary, the former combatants, when compared to the noncombatants, showed little or no evidence of the features of construing that might be thought to be associated with post-traumatic stress. Indeed, their views of themselves were particularly favourable, and they tended to see themselves

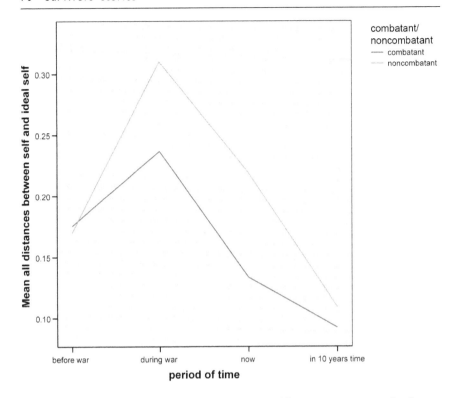

*Figure 5.1* Distances of self from how I should be at different points in time for former combatants and noncombatants. From Goins, S., Winter, D., Sundin, J., Patient, S., & Aslan, E. (2012). Self-construing in former child soldiers. *Journal of Constructivist Psychology, 25,* 275–301. Reprinted by permission of the publisher (Taylor & Francis Ltd, http://www.tandfonline.com).

now as better people than they had ever been in their lives, and anticipated that they would become better still. How could this be? One possibility is that they were able to contrast themselves with their very negatively con-strued rebel commanders and to disavow responsibility for their actions dur-ing the war by taking the view that they were just obeying orders while under extreme duress, including the threat of death if they disobeyed. A further consideration is that during the war they had, in effect, fulfilled the role of 'young warriors' in apprenticeship with, and fostered by, powerful authority figures in the form of their commanding officers. Such a role is institution-alized in Sierra Leone, for example in secret society training, and so it may be that they felt little dislodgement from their core roles or from the roles perceived to be expected of them by others, and therefore little guilt or shame as defined by personal construct theory (Kelly, 1955; McCoy, 1981). Finally, the responsibility and power that they were given during the war contrasted with the powerlessness of most children in Sierra Leone (where it is said that 'pikin a pikin', a child is a child and not responsible for his or her actions). This power, including in some cases taking positions of authority over adults, may have boosted their self-esteem.

The favourable self-constructions of the female former combatants in the displacement camp, despite their experiences as both victims (inclusive invariably of rape) and perpetrators of violence, merits particular consideration. It may be that their perceived commonality with other camp residents fostered group cohesiveness, which was conducive to high self-esteem, similarly to reports of the effects of group therapy approaches with survivors of childhood sexual abuse (Harter & Neimeyer, 1995). Such commonality may have been particularly important in a situation in which they reported experiences of rejection and ridicule by females who had not been combatants. Also noteworthy was the tightness of their construing, which limited the extent to which they experienced conflict and therefore minimized anxiety. This seems consistent with comments that they made about how important it was to 'keep the mind occupied' and 'keep the mind from being idle'.

### Examples of individual grids

Averaged grid data cannot, of course, fully reflect the construing of individual research participants. However, a closer examination of the grids of some of the former combatants throws further light upon the issues with which they were faced. For example, the plot derived from the principal components analysis of the grid of Sorie,[47] whose story began this chapter, indicates his extremely negative construal of the rebel leader and himself during the war, contrasting with how he would like to, and should, be, and how he imagines that he will be in 10 years time (see Figure 5.2). While he sees himself as having moved since the war towards how he was before he was abducted, he considers that he is still some distance from his ideal self. The grid also revealed a dilemma in that he does not wish to be *controlled* (perhaps largely because of his experiences of being controlled in the rebel forces) but views people who are *not under control* (perhaps like the rebel commanders) as *bad, wild, disobedient, not trustworthy*, and *guilty*.[48] He may therefore consider that, were he to be less controlled, he would run the risk of moving in the direction of these latter, undesirable characteristics.

A similar picture of a very negative construal of a rebel commander and of herself during the war can be seen in the plot from the principal components analysis of a former female child soldier[49] (Figure 5.3) who, as reported earlier in the chapter, was abducted by the rebels and raped. In her case, a dilemma was that while she saw herself as someone who *suffers* but the person she should be as someone who *enjoys*, she construed people who enjoy as *ungrateful, bad*, and likely to *take revenge*,[50] all of which are characteristics that she would not want. Perhaps for her it was better to suffer than to experience enjoyment and risk becoming like the rebel soldiers whose hedonism she had associated with 'badness' during the war.

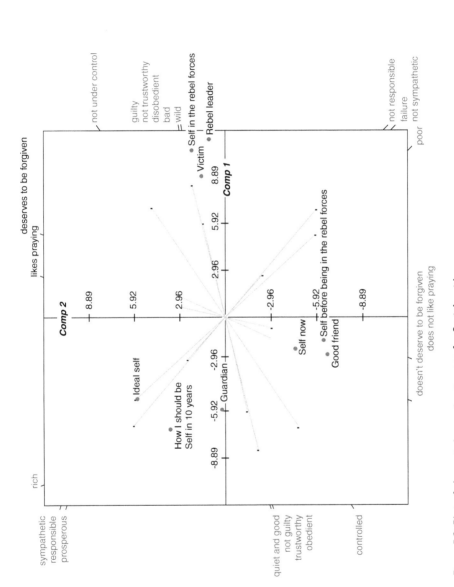

*Figure 5.2* Plot of elements in construct space for Sorie's grid

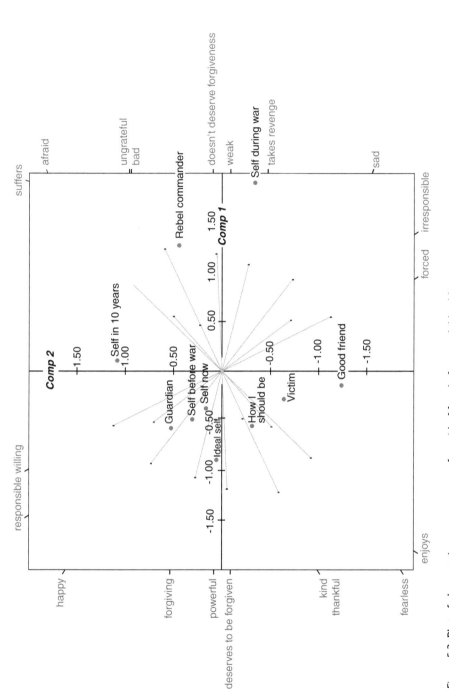

*Figure 5.3* Plot of elements in construct space for grid of female former child soldier

## Conclusions

The stories in this chapter depict the life of children caught up in fighting a war that they did not start, and that they would not have fought in, had circumstances been different. Sorie's phrase – *the saddest day of my life* – expressed a sentiment shared by all in Stephanie's data pool. The disruption of normal life, the dashed hopes, the annihilation of family and community, the extreme experiences of violence, all would seem to lead to the basic destruction of the human person, the soul as it were. Yet, we find an ability to withstand such destruction and even to overcome. Such is the resilience of the human spirit, a resilience that defies logic. This same resilience will be seen in the next chapter, where the stories of amputees and the reconstruction of life are examined.

## Notes

1  Interviewee #12.
2  Sorie had chosen not to take part in a secret society, because he and his family are practising Christians. They viewed some of the practices within this society as demonic and a compromise to their values. The actions he was forced to commit during his time with the RUF were as well, as will be seen later in this chapter.
3  This was not unusual. Interviewee #29 told me her daughter had been abducted by the RUF and was found after a year. She never asked her daughter for details about that time away.
4  Repeatedly in their narratives, former child soldiers shared these same deep and conflicting feelings.
5  Many former child soldiers from Stephanie's data pool expressed these same sentiments.
6  These can be found in the Appendix.
7  Again, see the Appendix.
8  *Afraid – fearless* has to do with authority and hierarchy. The one who is afraid is respectful of authority and hierarchy. The one who is fearless is not governed by respect for authority or hierarchical structure. In other words, his or her actions may fall into line with authority *if* s/he so chooses, but s/he is not ruled by fear of consequences for incompliance.
9  *Responsible – not responsible* has to do with being responsible for the care of someone or not, a construct that applies to (growing into) adulthood. *Responsible* is being accountable (caring) for someone or having another accountable (caring) for oneself. *Not responsible* would be the opposite situation, as in when children would write, 'I have no one to be responsible for me.'
10  *Powerful – weak* speaks of one's perception of power or control over a situation or circumstances. Similar to *suffers – enjoys*, this construct had to do with the war and its effects.
11  Those who wish to read more about repertory grids and their analysis are referred to Fransella, Bell and Bannister (2004) and Bell (2016).
12  #8, 14-year-old male, former soldier.
13  The situation for these boys was made worse by the fact that some teachers were prejudiced against them, it being obvious that the boys were former soldiers.
14  Interviewee #26. Momoh and the Community Theatre Agency he cofounded will be discussed in Chapter 13.
15  #17.
16  #9.
17  In Sierra Leone, the Mammy Queen (or Mummy Queen) is an elected position, a social institution, and was a recognized position of power and status for women.

According to several interviewees, women who fill this role mobilize other women for particular causes or purposes within a village or community. Mammy Queens are typically leaders of female secret societies, instrumental in rituals and ceremonies within those societies, and may serve as chiefs within some ethnic groups (Goins, 2015; McKay & Mazurana, 2004). In the war, the Mammy Queen was in charge of the females in the camp and would discipline the females if they did not obey the men. She also had the authority (and reputation) to force recruits into sexual relations with her, according to #28.

18  Interviewee #6. When Stephanie spoke with this Mende boy, he was 14 years old. He was at an interim care centre, and staff were trying to locate his family. The centre's director was extremely protective of this boy, who had been subjected to eight years of violence under the RUF.

19  #60.

20  RT, an 18-year-old female former soldier from a province, living in Freetown at the time of the January 1999 invasion. She was 15 years old at the time.

21  AB, 18-year-old female former soldier who was abducted at 15 years old.

22  #19, a 15-year-old female former soldier.

23  FM, 21 years old at the time of this recording; from a focus group in the Cline Town IDP camp, 14 February 2002.

24  #14.

25  #22.

26  #11, abducted and with the RUF for three years.

27  #28. Sadly, this girl was being used by her aunt, who was assistant principal, and ready to utilize whomever or whatever she could for personal gain. The girl was called into the office and was instructed to pull down the front of her dress so as to reveal the tattoo. The girl was asked to do this in the presence of Stephanie and Stephanie's male translator, both of whom she had never met.

28  This is not dissimilar to practices in other groups and regimes which have destroyed traditional community and family structures and involved children in brutal and oppressive acts. For example, the Khmer Rouge, followers of the Angkar or Communist Party of Cambodia, asserted that 'The *Angkar* is the mother and father of all young children, as well as all adolescent boys and girls' (Locard, 2004, p. 107, italics in original).

29  #18.

30  #61, a 15-year-old male former soldier who had been abducted.

31  Interviewee #5. Father Chema is a Xaverian priest and had lived in Sierra Leone for several years when Stephanie met him. His insights were invaluable. For a somewhat recent interview of Chema, see http://www.uoc.edu/portal/en/campus_pau/entrevistes/ent revistes/chema_caballero.html.

32  Interviewee #30.

33  Cline Town IDP camp residents told Stephanie this.

34  $t = 1.07$, ns

35  $F = 9.71, p < 0.01$ and $2.92, p < 0.10$ respectively

36  Wilks Lambda $= 0.77, F (3, 30) = 3.06, p < 0.05$

37  $F (1, 28) = 8.41, p < 0.01$

38  Wilks Lambda $= 0.30, F (3, 30) = 23.74, p < 0.001$

39  $p < 0.01$ and $< 0.001$, respectively

40  $p < 0.05$

41  combatants $p < 0.01$; noncombatants $p < 0.001$

42  combatants $p < 0.001$; noncombatants $p < 0.05$

43  $t = 1.84, p < 0.10$

44  $t = 2.38, p < 0.05$ and $1.91, p < 0.10$ respectively

45  $t = 1.82, p < 0.10$ and $4.59, p < 0.001$ respectively

46  $t = 2.48, p < 0.05$

47  Sorie's grid was completed during the pilot study, and the constructs in it were elicited from him rather than supplied, as was the case with the other participants.
48  As indicated by correlations between the construct '*controlled – not under control*' and the other constructs of 0.80, 0.61, 0.80, 0.80, and 0.80 respectively.
49  #19, 15 years old.
50  All correlations 0.51.

## References

Abraham, A. (2001) Dancing with the chameleon: Sierra Leone and the elusive quest for peace. *Journal of African Studies,* 19(2): 206–228.

Bell, R. C. (2009) *GRIDSTAT, version 5: A program for analyzing the data of a repertory grid* (computer software). Department of Psychology, University of Melbourne.

Bell, R. C. (2016) Methodologies of assessment in personal construct psychology. In D. A. Winter, N. Reed, *Wiley handbook of personal construct psychology.* Chichester: Wiley-Blackwell.

Bennett, A. (2002) *The reintegration of child ex-combatants in Sierra Leone with particular focus on the needs of females.* Unpublished MA, University of East London, London.

Boyden, J. (2003) The moral development of child soldiers: What do adults have to fear? *Peace and Conflict: Journal of Peace Psychology,* 9(4): 343–362.

deBoeck, P. (1986) *HICLAS computer program (version 1.0).* Leuven, Belgium: University of Leuven.

Feixas, G., Cornejo, J. M. (2002) *A manual for the repertory grid.* Available at: http://www.terapiacognitiva.net/record/pag/man10.htm [Accessed 17 January 2005].

Finnegan, R. (1964) 'Swears' among the Limba. *The Sierra Leone Bulletin of Religion,* 6(1): 8–25.

Fransella, F., Bell, R., Bannister, D. (2004) *A manual for repertory grid technique* (2nd ed.). Chichester: Wiley.

Gbla, O. (2003) Conflict and post-war trauma among child soldiers in Liberia and Sierra Leone. In A. Sesay (Ed.), *Civil wars, child soldiers and post conflict peace building in West Africa* (pp. 167–194). Ibadan, Nigeria: Nigerian College Press Publishers.

Goins, S. (2015) *Forgiveness and reintegration: How the transformative process of forgiveness impacts child soldier reintegration* (provisional title). Oxford: Regnum Books.

Goins, S., Winter, D., Sundin, J., Patient, S., Aslan, E. (2012) Self construing in former child soldiers. *Journal of Constructivist Psychology,* 25: 275–301.

Govier, T. (2006) *Taking wrongs seriously: Acknowledgment, reconciliation, and the politics of sustainable peace.* Amherst, NY: Humanity Books.

Grice, J. (2002) Idiogrid: Software for the management and analysis of repertory grids. *Behavior Research Methods, Instruments, & Computers,* 34: 338–341.

Harter, S. L., Neimeyer, R. A. (1995) Long term effects of child sexual abuse: Toward a constructivist theory of trauma and its treatment. In R. A. Neimeyer, G. J. Neimeyer (Eds.), *Advances in personal construct psychology* (Vol. 3, pp. 229–269). Greenwich, CT: JAI Press.

HRW (Human Rights Watch) (2001) *Sexual violence within the Sierra Leone conflict.* Available at: http://pantheon.hrw.org/legacy/backgrounder/africa/sl-bck0226.htm [Accessed 17 January 2005].

Kelly, G. A. (1955) *The psychology of personal constructs.* New York: Norton. (Reprinted by Routledge, 1991)

Locard, H. (2004) *Pol Pot's little red book: The sayings of Angkar.* Chiang Mai: Silkworm Books.

Lowicki, J., Pillsbury, A. A. (2002) *Precious resources: Adolescents in the reconstruction of Sierra Leone.* New York: Women's Commission for Refugee Women and Children.

McCoy, M. (1981) Positive and negative emotions. In H. Bonarius, R. Holland, S. Rosenberg (Eds.), *Personal construct psychology: Recent advances in theory and practice* (pp. 95–104). New York: St. Martin's Press.

McKay, S., Mazurana, D. (2004) *Where are the girls? Girls in fighting forces in Northern Uganda, Sierra Leone and Mozambique: Their lives during and after war.* Montreal: International Centre for Human Rights and Democratic Development.

Orley, J. (1976) The use of grid technique in social anthropology. In P. Slater (Ed.), *The measurement of intrapersonal space by grid technique. Vol. 1: Explorations of intrapersonal space* (pp. 219–232). Chichester: Wiley.

Peters, K., Richards, P. (1998) Fighting with open eyes: Young combatants talking about war in Sierra Leone. In P.C.P. Bracken (Ed.), *Rethinking the trauma of war* (pp. 76–111). London: Free Association Books.

Veale, A. (2003) *From child soldier to ex-fighter: female fighters, demobilization, and reintegration in Ethiopia. Monograph No. 85.* Pretoria: Institute for Security Studies.

Voeten, T. (2000) *How de body?* (R. Vatter-Buck, Trans.). New York: St. Martin's Press.

Zack-Williams, A. B. (2001) Child soldiers in the civil war in Sierra Leone. *Review of African Political Economy* 28(87): 73–82.

# Chapter 6

# Amputees' stories

## Reconstructing life as a one-foot person

There is no better way of beginning a Saturday morning in Freetown than to walk along the idyllic stretch of sand that is Lumley Beach. Admittedly, this is hardly a place for peace and solitude. You will have to negotiate a few scraggy dogs and the occasional vulture scavenging amongst whatever the sea has deposited during the night. You may lend a hand to fishermen bringing in their catch. You will be passed by a succession of joggers who appear to be approaching their exercise as earnestly as their work with the plethora of NGOs that operate in Freetown. You will be asked, and will find it hard to refuse, to buy jewellery fashioned out of shells and stones, or carvings, or batik. You will be engaged in conversations, which may lead to the prospect of more substantial purchases: diamonds, perhaps, or introductions to young women. The sound of the waves is certain to be accompanied by the strains of music – probably African reggae – which is ever-present in Sierra Leone.

It will also be no surprise to hear shouts and see in the distance people playing football, since this is no less a passion in Sierra Leone than elsewhere in Africa. Cars, trucks, and boats generally either carry religious messages (e.g., God bless Allah; His only Son) or the names of English Premier League football teams (e.g., Da Gunners – the nickname of Arsenal Football Club), and sometimes both (e.g., on a fishing boat: Have Faith in God . . . Winners . . . Liverpool), and large crowds gather around and peer through cracks in the walls of shacks in which live screenings of football matches, again mostly from England, are shown. However, on walking towards the football players on the beach, you will begin to make out that, although fast and furious, something about the players' movement indicates that theirs is no ordinary game. This is because what you will have stumbled upon is the weekly practice session of the Sierra Leone Single-Leg Amputee Football Club.[1] All its outfield players have one leg and its goalkeepers have one arm, and all lost their limbs during the civil war. Their stories, which will be told in this chapter, exemplify the horror and resilience that are characteristic of their country.

### The terror of amputation

Although you may only occasionally encounter amputee footballers, you will see many amputees in Freetown. One reason for this is that, during the civil war, amputation was one of the favourite forms of terror used by the rebel soldiers.

Their victims would typically be given a choice, but this would be between 'long sleeves' and 'short sleeves', namely having one's arms amputated at the wrist or at the elbow.[2] The amputation would often be presented as a punishment for the victim having used their arm and hand to vote for the government, and to ensure that they would not do so again. They would also often be told that they should ask the government to provide them with new (prosthetic) limbs. Legs were amputated as well as arms, and sometimes victims were deliberately shot in one of their legs, causing such destruction that it then had to be medically amputated.

While media reports and cinematic portrayals of atrocities such as this often carried the (at least implicit) message that they represented a uniquely African barbarism, the extent to which they differed in their savagery from acts committed in wars anywhere else in the globe is arguable.[3] It is also worth bearing in mind that amputation as a form of terror was practised in Africa by its colonial masters long before the civil war in Sierra Leone.[4]

## Research methods

Interviews were conducted with 32 amputee footballers[5] on two visits to Freetown. Their ages ranged from 11 to 40 years, with a mean age of 26.52 years. The age at which they lost their limbs ranged from to 1 to 27 years, with a mean age of 13.13 years. All except one were male.

In view of Sierra Leone's rich oral story-telling tradition, it was considered that an interview requesting a narrative account of participants' experiences would be an appropriate method of data collection (Manganyi, 1991). An audio-taped interview was therefore conducted, with each participant asked the questions outlined in Table 6.1 (although, in the interests of narrative flow, not always in the order presented). Consistent with the principal concerns of personal construct theory (Kelly, 1955), the interview attempted to explore participants' construing of their past, present, and future; the choices considered to be open (or closed) to them; and their *sociality*, or understanding of the views and actions, of those responsible for their predicaments (Winter, 2015).

Twenty-five of the participants also completed a repertory grid (see Chapter 5) in which the elements were *me now; me before the war; me during the war before I lost a limb; me during the war after I lost a limb; me in 10 years time; me when playing football; how I would like to be; the person responsible for my injury now; the person responsible for my injury before the war; the person responsible for my injury during the war; the person responsible for my injury in 10 years time; amputee football team players;* and *a normal person.* Participants rated these elements on a 7-point scale on the following constructs, which were derived from the interviews with the first nine participants (representing common themes in these interviews): *happy – miserable; discouraged – has hope; in pain – not in pain; good – wicked; does not have problems – has problems; has no support – has support; doesn't suffer – suffers; has no way to earn money – has a way to earn money; proud – not proud; not respected – respected; lonely – not lonely; forgiving – not forgiving.*

*Table 6.1* Interview schedule with amputee footballers

| |
| --- |
| *I would like to hear your life story, from childhood to how you are now.* |
| *How old were you when you lost your limb?* |
| *Why do you think they did this?* |
| *What do you feel about the people who were responsible?* |
| *What would you want to say to them if you met them?* |
| *How do you think your life would have been if this had not happened to you?* |
| *How do you see the future?* |
| *What sort of things make you feel better?* |
| *How does football make a difference to you?* |
| *Is there anything else you want to say?* |

## Interview responses

### Loss of limbs

Although not specifically asked to do so, virtually all of the participants began their accounts with a description of the incidents that had led to the loss of their limbs, as if these constituted the beginning of the current stories of their lives (Winter and Wood, 2012). These incidents primarily involved arms or legs being amputated by the rebel soldiers. In some instances, a leg or foot was deliberately destroyed by gunfire and subsequently amputated, either by the rebels or medically in those who were fortunate enough to be rescued and taken to hospital. In one or two cases, limbs were also lost in explosions during the war.

A typical scenario was as follows:

> *They make three lines, one for the children, one for the fathers and one for the girls, the women, our mothers. After that they took all the men behind the wall of the house in the compound and later we started hearing gunshots. So they took our mothers away, they put them in their vehicles to go with them and we, the children, they said we are coming to cut our feet. So unfortunately they start, I'm the second child. I'm the second person in my compound to be amputated.*
>
> [F24, aged 24, amputated aged 6][6]

The amputation was often presented as a punishment for not providing information that the rebels demanded, for refusing to join them, or for presumed support of the government. For example:

> *they said they don't want to kill me, but they're going to punish me and that's why they punish me, they shoot my leg.*
>
> [F15, aged 27, amputated aged 8]

> *... during the war I was caught by the rebels in Freetown in 1999 and they chop off my hand without doing nothing with them. I don't know nothing about this war, how the war came to Sierra Leone but I would suffer. They chopped off my hand.*

*They wanted to know about the ECOMOG soldiers and they go to our house in Freetown and they asked us about the ECOMOG soldiers. We told them that we don't know about them because we are civilians. So we are pleading with them for them not to shoot us . . . and suddenly . . . they started to get violent . . . in the house. My hand was cut off.*

[F26, aged 28, amputated aged 15]

*They came to town and . . . by then they need more young men to join them so they captured me. I refused to join them so that's when they decided to cut off my leg. They cut off my leg, and I was suffering, suffering, suffering.*

[F22, aged 31, amputated aged 17]

When an 11-year-old boy and his friends had no food to give to the rebels, their response was as follows:

*So they say we are going to cut off your hand and then the Sierra Leone government is going to give you a hand. . . . We said no, it is not fair, why do you treat us like this? They asked us to go to a line, they said we are going to cut your hands. . . . They tie our arms behind our backs. A long stick and water on our bodies, glug, glug, glug. About 4 of my friends they cut their two arms. We are one side. I said OK, I can't believe you do this. 5 of us they cut one arm.*

[F16, aged 24, amputated aged 11]

In several instances, the amputation was accompanied by the additional horror of witnessing the murder or rape of family members. For example:

*They have beat my father . . . until dead. . . . They had ask me for my father property, my father money . . . I told them that I young boy, I don't know how my father keep money. And after that they have start to beat me . . . one RF boy brought weapon – fire me in my foot, about 3 shots. . . . My foot finish for, cut off.*

[F5, aged 26, amputated aged 16]

*I met the rebels and they asked us everyone get out of the car and get down, when we get down, they put us together and my father, they shot my father, they shoot him and some of us around them they shot them and they cut off our legs.*

[F27, aged 24, amputated aged 12]

*At that time the rebels catch me, they chopped, they chopped my leg at that time, they caught all my family too, they raped my mother, they killed my father, at that time they shot my father down, they killed my father. They said OK, you. We have something to do to you, come here. They took my leg and chopped it, they chopped my leg.*

[F23, aged 27, amputated aged 13]

*I was 5 years old. I was with my family. They catch my mother, they catch my father, my grandmother. . . . They took us, the people, and they started firing. They shoot some of them, they chop some of them, some of us, chop some of their hands, they chop arms, they chop legs, they cut heads, the neck, at that time we were not sure and I was like a baby, I was crying, crying. They killed my mother, they took me from my mother, they took me and they started chopping my leg and they leave me there where they chop my leg and they leave me. I started crying, I started crying, I started crying.*

[F18, aged 31, amputated aged 5]

*I was 12 in 1999. I lost my right hand, they go and cut it, after that I had to use the other hand. They had to cut it down. They rape my mother, she was trying to help me, my mother said 'no' . . . my Dad. After they cut it, they warned me relax, my mother watching, she died, she get fed up watching me, she died.*

[F13, aged 24, amputated aged 12]

Many people died of their wounds, for example from tetanus, in the bush because they were unable to receive medical attention. However, even if they did manage to get taken to hospital, this did not necessarily provide any relief. As one participant described:

*The hospital was totally empty, all the medical staff, even the doctors and nurses had run away. They are not at the hospital. So I had a shot leg with no proper medication.*

[F32, aged 24, amputated aged 10]

Although in this case the staff did eventually return, so did the rebels to inflict yet more terror on the amputees:

*. . . they came around the beds and asking us why were we amputated, are we happy. Then most . . . of the people who said they were not happy they shot them again so they were killed and some of the other people who were taking care of us, like my elder sister were killed at that time. . . . Even those who were not happy, they ask you what form of amputation do you want, is it a long leg or a short leg.*

[F32, aged 24, amputated aged 10]

### Searching for meaning

All of the participants struggled to find any meaning in what had happened to them. In attempting to show sociality (Kelly, 1955), or see the world through the eyes of their assailants, they were only able to conclude that the perpetrators did it 'because they felt like doing it' or 'for nothing', since they did not know their victims, for example:

*They did it because they just feel like doing it to them.*

[F6, aged 38, amputated aged 27][7]

*He never knew them, he don't have no experience about these people, they just shot him for nothing.*

[F9, aged 11, amputated aged 1]

*He was a civilian. He was not doing anything, he was not a soldier, he was not a policeman, and they shot him.*

[F20, aged 40, amputated aged 14]

*Why did the rebels do that? I don't know anything. We don't know the reason why they're attacking for. The reason why the rebels started the war in Sierra Leone, we don't know the reason.*

[F28, aged 29, amputated aged 10]

*Actually, I don't know. I don't know why. I'm not part of the war. I'm not a soldier neither. I don't know why they do that.*

[F27, aged 22, amputated aged 12]

*I was a little boy. So, I don't know. I don't know why. I am not part of government, I don't know the government, I don't know why, I don't know they shot my leg. Up to this day I don't know.*

[F19, aged 34, amputated aged 14]

Although some amputees were able to explain something of the context of the civil war, for example in terms of the rebels receiving arms from Liberia in return for 'blood diamonds', they still could not understand why the rebels should then use these weapons to shoot and kill people without the people having done anything to deserve this. This seemed particularly hard to understand when their assailants were small boys:

*It's because of these blood diamonds that we have . . . they travelled from Liberia and came along with weapons . . . they . . . hand over these weapons to these guys in the bush and they took diamonds from them. So these guys, they went on the street just to shoot people and kill them without doing anything. You see this small boy like this, without no government or anything like that, just see us, when moving he shot us.*

[F8, aged 26, amputated aged 18]

*Why? Because of the diamonds and other things that are in this country, that's why. No reason. When you ask them, they say we are the people suffering too much in this country. Our father is a member of parliament. We say no, our father is not a member of parliament. They say your father is living in Kono and he has diamonds, that's why we do anything we want to do to you at that time.*

[F23, aged 27, amputated aged 13]

*I don't know who is responsible for this particular war. I don't know whether it's the government or the people . . . supplying them with arms and ammunition. Liberia gives them the knowledge, the skills how to do it. I think it's the government, I don't know who is responsible for supplying.*

[F32, aged 24, amputated aged 10]

*Well, when I was young I used to be confused about these rebels because I was not even grown up. The government was in disarray. There was political . . . this government was having problems keeping control and the war has to come. From my understanding, I never know what is the problem because . . . I know that like the government, they say that the government is causing the war but how can this be . . . because after the war we have a president Kabbah put an end to the war so how can this government if it is causing this war bring an end to this war?*

[F31, aged 20, amputated aged 7]

*There is no reason, they told me no reason. By then when I was getting old now at the age of 12 I still remember so I called my father and asked why did the people do this to me so my father said the question you ask is a rhetorical question. So he will not answer, he will not answer, he will not do anything. So it's just an offence. By then I was hearing people saying that just because of political powers, political influence it was between two different parties. So I asked my father which party did you support at that time. He didn't tell me. He didn't tell me at that time.*

[F21, aged 22, amputated aged 6]

### Loss of opportunities

The participants described not only losing their limbs but also consequently educational, occupational, and romantic opportunities, and more generally the ability to live a normal life:

*While he is amputated he has no way to get money to survive.*

[F6, aged 38, amputated aged 27]

*If you don't have money you don't have anybody that will help you. You don't have anybody that will come to your aid, that will help you, you'll be like that something that will be thrown away in the dustbin nobody will want so really that's how it is . . . in our country if you are deformed nobody will help you, nobody will take care of you because out there they want everyone to work for our daily bread.*

[F32, aged 24, amputated aged 10]

*If he want a woman . . . he can't give her money. I think the love can't extend, it cannot go further. . . .*

[F4, aged 37, amputated aged 15]

*When he was not amputated, he was living normal life, now he's not living normal life, the way he was before.*

[F7, aged 27, amputated aged 18]

*Sometimes I will feel discouraged because presently I don't have no support to even continue my education.*

[F2, aged 33, amputated aged 18]

### Guilt and shame

Their lost opportunities led participants to be dislodged from their core under-standing of their roles in life, an experience that Kelly (1955) equated with guilt. For example:

*What I was doing before I'm not able to do it . . . land a job . . . most of the people will not take me back.*

[F2, aged 33, amputated aged 18]

Participants were also dislodged from others' views of their core roles, which McCoy (1977) has equated with the experience of shame. Thus, many of them described the negative reactions of others to their disabilities, for example:

*The whole village, I'm the only one who have this problem, all of them there they are capable, so even that I go to the village . . . I cannot feel any good.*

[F5, aged 26, amputated aged 16]

*If I stand alone waiting for a vehicle to take me back home, they won't stop. They say you're amputated. They don't care. They say you don't have money to pay. They say leave me alone. I stand there for 4 hours . . . because amputees are not respected in my country here.*

[F8, aged 26, amputated aged 18]

*Because they have two legs, two hands, but today I have one leg. I'm not happy because everywhere I go some people laugh me, they say look at one-leg man, they say look at the one-leg man, that's how some people laugh me or call me. But still I appreciate that today I have one leg still good.*

[F15, aged 27, amputated aged 8]

*They see with one foot, they not respect me . . . they don't pity a one-foot man.*

[F3, aged 29, amputated aged 15]

For this participant, the lack of respect also included how his children might view him if he were to become a father:

*They not go be proud of you . . . mama lives with hand cut or me papa lives with foot cut.*

[F3, aged 29, amputated aged 15]

### Anxiety

In Kelly's (1955) view, when one finds it hard to construe events, one experiences anxiety. Many of the amputees not only found it hard to make sense of what had happened to them in the civil war but also found it hard to envisage the future, which was therefore a source of considerable anxiety. For example:

> *Well my future I find it difficult because I believe even the able people in the world . . . all over the world, or Freetown, Sierra Leone they find it difficult for them to live, so I – what about me when I lost my leg, so how am I going to get my future plan?*
>
> [F4, aged 37, amputated aged 15]

> *Well, sometimes when I think about my amputation I lose hope. When I think about my amputation . . . our country is hard even for the able bodied to survive. When I am thinking about that I think how can I be able to survive? The able bodied it is too hard for them to earn their living. What about me, who is disabled? So I find it difficult.*
>
> [F24, aged 24, amputated aged 6]

> *I hope the future will be better but it's not easy, in Africa it's not easy. In Africa we are always crying for people to help us, especially the amputees. The war-affected amputees, we lost a lot, we lost many people, we lost housing, we lost our relatives, we lost a lot, even our hope and our lives, we just think . . . we have a little bit hope but not much.*
>
> [F19, aged 34, amputated aged 14]

### Strategies for survival

#### Avoidance of anxiety, guilt, and shame

One of the amputees avoided anxiety about the future because he saw constant rumination about what might happen as paradoxically itself causing one to lose one's present life:

> *Yeh, it's like not going to anxious again because as soon as I lost my leg I shall not watch anything because if I watch my life I shall lose my life, so that's why I just take things easy.*
>
> [F14, aged 36, amputated aged 19]

This individual was also able to see the amputation as merely the loss of a limb and not necessarily of other aspects of his life and roles. For example:

> *. . . when I lost my leg it's not nice, I don't lost, it's not opportunities I lost, only my legs I lost, it's not the ending of my life yeh? When there is life I know there is hope*

*so that's why I'm happy when you are here, when you're going to interview us, the football guys, so we are glad.*

[F14, aged 36, amputated aged 19]

For some people, a strategy such as this involved contrasting themselves with other amputees who had been less fortunate:

*Although I'm an amputee I'm still living. This is why . . . like meeting with you today. If I'm not alive I'm not able to do it but see, I'm alive.*

[F32, male aged 24, amputated aged 10]

*Plenty of them, they're out of their heads now because of the pains.*

[F1, age unknown, amputated aged 15]

*Some people has died because of this problem. Most of my friends, because of the pain they die in hospital.*

[F2, aged 33, amputated aged 18]

*I have friends, amputees, and they could die any year because . . . tetanus . . . they not able to recover from that sickness except their dying from that thing.*

[F3, aged 29, amputated aged 15]

## Dependency on God

A very common response to any difficulty in Sierra Leone is to 'leave it to God', often abrogating any sense of personal agency. Such a strategy was apparent in the accounts of several of the amputees, for example:

*If God helps him to have money, he will enjoy himself by doing business so that he can support his family.*

[F7, aged 27, amputated aged 18]

*He's feeling bad, he's not feeling good, at times when he wake up he feel abnormal because of his amputation, and he leaves his case to God, for God to take care of everything.*

[F6, aged 38, amputated aged 27]

*You have to bear and put your trust to God, the hope, likewise encourage yourself, pray to God for Him to control you as He wants, not what you want.*

[F1, age unknown, amputated aged 15]

*Well, my future is with God because He made everything possible for so my future is with God. That's why I used to go to church and pray so that my future get brighter, so that I will not be worried in the future.*

[F27, aged 24, amputated aged 12]

*I would only say that it's only God . . . God puts you in this place. God says I need to be an amputee. I was amputated, I was amputated, yes.*

[F15, aged 27, amputated aged 8]

### Earning money

Some of the participants saw their only means of survival as joining the armies of beggars on the streets of Freetown, although this often increased their sense of guilt and shame, for example:

*Now he find a way to have money, every day he go to the street and beg.*

[F7, aged 27, amputated aged 18]

*He's walking along the street every day. When people see him they give him money, but that one is not good.*

[F9, aged 11, amputated aged 1]

However, one or two had either pursued their education or been able to find employment, and in one case, the participant viewed his present state as even better than it had been prior to his amputation:

*By now living better than before the time I was having the problem so now I'm try-ing to do some studies so that may the Lord help me to achieve most things in my life, actually but now I'm technicians for me not to be on the street . . . so as from now I'm living in good conditions because there is a life and I hope there is a hope.*

[F1, age unknown, amputated aged 15]

## Recovery through football

Whatever else contributed to their recovery, it was apparent that football played a major role in this, and that there were several aspects to this process.

### Reducing guilt and shame

First, football led to the reduction of guilt and shame, allowing amputees to regain both self-respect and the perceived respect of others by demonstrating that they should not just be viewed as beggars but that they are able to do some-thing that able-bodied people can do.

As the founder of the team had explained it to the rather dubious amputees whom he persuaded to join:

*They killed my mother, killed my father, and my sister so I'm from the province, I came in the city. When I came I met my companions, I made them, all, every one of them, start tell their problems. I tried to become president for the amputees, so*

*I tried to decide, I tried to decide. I said 'You guys, never mind we lost our legs, some of us lost our hands, we're not anything in the sight of God, we're not the ones who make us, so let's come together and decide to play football'. So some of them have doubts, say 'We have no legs so how can we play football?' I say 'No, I will go out and do it for you guys to just to watch me and you can follow.' So I decide, I take these guys over two months, I try to train them, training them, training them, training them until these guys became perfect in the soccer play. They tell us to go the province to play there, to organize there just to show people never mind we lost our legs still we can do what people able can do so we go there, we train, we played some games, people came out and watch us, so after that we came back.*

[F14, aged 36, amputated aged 19]

This vision of the benefits of playing football was validated by the accounts of several of the amputees, for example:

*For do something . . . other man can when they go play ball when one – two – thousand people they go watch you.*

[F3, aged 29, amputated aged 15]

*. . . when I think about football I think about joy . . . because we too can play like the able, I can play very well. I have strength and health too. They give you courage.*

[F16, aged 24, amputated aged 11]

*(playing football) make my life feel proud for now because while I play football, I forget everything.*

[F5, aged 26, amputated aged 16]

*he's glad because when people see them along the street at times they class them to be beggars but they are telling them that they play football internationally they are not beggars . . . never mind that they are amputated, but they can do something that able man can do.*

[F6, aged 38, amputated aged 27]

*People come to me, they've heard about me. . . . Everybody knows about me. When I walk along the street they say . . . [participant's name], oh. . . .*

[F8, aged 26, amputated aged 18]

*I feel proud because I am in the amputee football team.*

[F9, aged 11, amputated aged 1]

*When I play football I courage myself so that is the only thing that make me happy. When I play soccer I forget about the past. Yes. I am one of the kings of the soccer.*

[F14, aged 36, amputated aged 19]

*Football in effect allowed team members to regain credibility in ourselves because we think that what everybody can do amputees like us can do that . . . and so by playing football we motivate ourselves, yeah. Football bring us together, so with football we achieve a lot, by going to England, to Brazil, you know, to Turkey, to Holland, so football has made us to achieve a lot. With two legs you cannot go there, but with one leg because I'm a player I've been there, so I appreciate a lot.*

[F8, aged 26, amputated aged 18]

### New opportunities

This quote also indicates another benefit that football provided, namely that it paradoxically gave opportunities, for example for travel, that would never have been available to them had they not lost their limbs. For some participants, this led them to regard their lives at present as better than they had ever been:

*I will see another things, I will see plenty things, get more idea, knowledge over the travelling in the world, now am so happy because of now I'm playing for single leg amputee sport club in Sierra Leone. I play so many competition. I've play competition since 2003 in England with the white amputee guys so likewise I play competition Turkey, Brazil and Russia, etc. so there was a success so that's why I say my life now is better.*

[F1, age unknown, amputated aged 15]

*You know, in life there is something that happens that creates another opportunity. If I'm not an amputee maybe I wouldn't have had the opportunity to travel abroad but being part of this team has made a lot of impact on me, you know exposing me to parts of the world worldwide. Some countries people know me there personally so India, Namibia, Tanzania, they say when are we going to have time. I don't have time.*

[F17, aged 25, amputated aged 10]

*Yes, my life has changed because of the amputation because we . . . go to different countries. . . . I have travelled to different countries.*

[F26, aged 28, amputated aged 15]

For some football team members, playing abroad not only offered new experiences but also temptations:

*These boys, they go to England, they go to Brazil, they go Paralympics . . . they go there for two weeks, and after the programme they come back and they're showing that they're proud of their country. But when you go to Europe they try to escape.*

[F6, aged 38, amputated aged 27]

### Comradeship

Another major beneficial aspect of football for the participants was the sense of commonality (Kelly, 1955), or a shared way of viewing the world, that it gave them with their fellow amputees. This is similar to the curative factor in group psychotherapy that Yalom (1970) terms 'universality', involving a 'welcome to the human race' experience. For example:

> *We join ourselves together to meet our interest . . . we feel happy, because we see ourselves together.*
>
> [F4, aged 37, amputated aged 15]

> *Well, one thing that makes me feel good is when I go to the beach and play with my friends who are disabled. We are all together, we chat, when I see my friends who are disabled I feel happy, I'm not thinking about my disability so I feel happy, especially when we have a trip to go to nationwide.*
>
> [F24, aged 24, amputated aged 6]

> *Well I would say that because I live with my brother amputees close together, I think that not me only amputee, there are amputees around the world and that's why my brother amputees, we discuss together, we make things together, we make fun together. Yes that's what makes us happy in my life, to see my brother amputees, that's what makes our happy.*
>
> [F15, aged 27, amputated aged 8]

> *(I have no one close to me) except my friends that we play football . . . because in Africa or Sierra Leone they love somebody because of, you know, money.*
>
> [F4, aged 37, amputated aged 15]

> *I cannot feel any good unless I be with my colleagues so that I feel good, yes, because them they are amputate, me I am amputate.*
>
> [F5, aged 26, amputated aged 16]

> *He was . . . lonely . . . now because he join these guys playing football he achieve new life that . . . they're friends.*
>
> [F6, aged 38, amputated aged 27]

> *I am with my friends together . . . on a Saturday, we come together, we play at the beach. . . . When I go, we laugh together, we talk together.*
>
> [F8, aged 26, amputated aged 18]

It was clear that the experience of playing football with other amputees gave participants a sense of courage, and made them feel that they had come alive again:

> *It make me . . . alive. They saved me. I was like a dropout and when I came to Freetown no one could give me the courage . . . like when I met them . . . when I*

*came to realize that . . . courage, like being in the team has given me more courage true to the fact other factors like socially, interactively, emotionally I've opened to see many things, and I've gained many knowledge.*

[F32, aged 24, amputated aged 10]

*. . . my life has changed because since when I joined the amputee football team my colleagues encouraged, they motivate me to play in competition, they advise me. At first when I always become sad, I don't have anyone to encourage me, to console me, to advise me, to motivate me, something like that.*

[F29, aged 31, amputated aged 16]

*. . . when you have amputation it is one of the most discouraging things in your life. The moment I started to move along with my colleagues who had the same problems as mine I started to take courage.*

[F19, aged 34, amputated aged 13]

*Well, when I am with my brother amputees, any time it gives courage, I am happy to be with my brother amputees so sometimes when we walk on the street I have only one arm I can help the others.*

[F16, aged 24, amputated aged 11]

Football not only allowed participants to experience commonality with their team members but also with the entire community:

*Well the football make a big difference to me because since . . . my problem I came that time out of the society or the community . . . but since we join ourselves together with the football club I believe that I be part of the community again because when they take us going to the different location or environment we have . . . the number of people watching us . . . so that show that we are still in the community.*

[F4, aged 37, amputated aged 15]

*Get inside the motor car with the whole . . . play different region . . . play with fun we even sing . . . other people who left the camp admire me because they know respect me.*

[F3, aged 29, amputated aged 15]

### Confronting the perpetrator

The people who had been responsible for the loss of the participants' limbs could well now be living freely in the community, most probably with less hardship than the participants, in part as a result of support provided by the government when they were demobilized. What would the participants want to say or do if they encountered them in the course of their daily lives?

Some wanted to communicate to the perpetrators the magnitude of the effects of their actions, and that they should now be responsible for taking care of the amputee:

> *Well I would just like to tell him that the thing he do to me I will not feeling well . . . but I will tell him my case to God . . . I will tell him that the thing he did to me spoil my future.*
>
> [F2, aged 33, amputated aged 18]

> *I will tell him that he should take care of all my abilities because I have so many problems in my life so that he can take care of all my responsibility in my life, so but I know not the very person in my life who did it, only the God almighty.*
>
> [F1, age unknown, amputated aged 15]

Only the youngest participant expressed any wish to take retaliatory action against the perpetrator:

> *I think to kill him or her.*
>
> [F9, aged 11, amputated aged 1]

In most cases, however, participants viewed the incident as having 'passed' and left it to God to address it:

> *I have nothing to do because it has already passed but I think that God has something for me because I lost my leg but since I am alive . . . if I see him, I always feel a fresh pain.*
>
> [F4, aged 37, amputated aged 15]

> *Leave him with God just leave him with God, I have nothing to do.*
>
> [F13, aged 24, amputated aged 12]

Although the people of Sierra Leone had been asked to adopt an attitude of 'forgive and forget' towards the events of the civil war, it was clear that this was not altogether easy for all of the amputees. The rather confused accounts of some of the participants perhaps indicated their conflict about this issue, or a discrepancy between what they felt and what they believed that they should say. These accounts included the following:

> *When the war ended the United Nations and the government said we have to forgive and forget. So we all know we have to forgive. To be frank, I have no, no feeling right now because I know everything that happened. I have no grudges. I have to forgive. The only thing is that trying to forgive is very difficult. Going out every day, coming across these people, so it's like very difficult walking on the streets of Freetown people watching you you get very aggressive sometimes because people watching you. You*

*know that something is wrong with you, that is why they are watching you. You forget, you try to forgive.*

[F31, aged 20, amputated aged 7]

*I don't feel good, I don't feel good now, now, now we have peace in this country let us forget. I forget but I don't forgive, I forget but I don't forgive but now because we want to have peace in this country I don't have no problem so now I only forgive, I never forget, that's why I never forget. . . . If I meet the person now I will just say if you are the person who make me to be chopping I don't have a chance to . . . I don't have that power if I had power I will chop your hand. I forgive you, I forgive you. That's why I say I will never forget.*

[F23, aged 27, amputated aged 13]

*Oh if I know him I will not do anything because I was told that I should forgive. Now I have forgiven but this is not, this is not something that can be forgotten because every time you see yourself as a cripple it is not something I should forget. You can only forgive in your heart but you cannot forget.*

[F21, aged 22, amputated aged 6]

*Forgive him? Well, in this world I cannot plan to look at . . . anything like what he did to me that's for God. Perhaps God will punish him according to what he did to me.*

[F28, aged 29, amputated aged 10]

*. . . I deh just control my heart, I . . . waiting God now. . . . You not deh forget but want forgive because where I feel the pain or where I see me mind effect . . . but I don't forgive them.*

[F3, aged 29, amputated aged 15]

Some of the participants' ability to forgive seemed to be associated with an attempt to show 'sociality' with the perpetrators, seeing the world through their eyes in an attempt to understand what they had done or their current situations, for example:

*He would forgive him. They were taking drugs, they don't know what they are doing, and he would forgive them.*

[F25, aged 15, amputated aged 3]

*The person that has done this to him, he might see him on the way going, it has nothing to do with him, because now he realise that he has a family.*

[F6, aged 38, amputated aged 27]

However, the commonest reason expressed for forgiveness and lack of retaliation against the perpetrators was that this was for the sake of peace in the amputees' country:

*Well if I see the person who shot me, I won't do anything you see because . . . my foot will not be properly again. So I just forgive him to God that everything is forgiven.*

*I will not do anything because we will have peace in our country, that's why I will think of peace.*

[F8, aged 26, amputated aged 18]

*For now I pray to God what . . . done happen with me for during the war, I pray for God that like that doesn't happen again in this country again.*

[F5, aged 26, amputated aged 16]

*Because, we have to peace so I just have to embrace him, we have to forgive and forget, so I'll forgive and forget about him.*

[F30, aged 20, amputated aged 8]

*Now? Now they are out from the bush, everybody getting peace so we all happy. We all like the president, Dr. Koroma, he try very hard because he bring peace and Kabbah . . . he brings the peace so that people, rebels these people all came out, and so now we're getting peace, they have elections, and so now we're always looking for this man. The honest President Koroma who try to all people to be one, to change their attitude so we always look up to the president because life will be stable to go give parliament in Freetown. So we have to say that the country is stable, without any kind of problem that will affect us so we appreciate that.*

[F11, aged 23, amputated aged 11]

*Neh, I want to forgive. They are my brothers, my sisters, so as for me you are supposed to get more experience from this kind of war so we are supposed to say the kind of country we find ourselves, Sierra Leone, we have everything. That's why when we are thinking about the development of Sierra Leone, we all want to say we are able to go forward and employ in a good job . . . like me, I need, I need to work, when you write the application and tell them you are handicapped, you are amputee, they are not happy always . . . when we are not happy we do bad stuff, so if people saw them they forgive and forget so we come together for improve for Sierra Leone this is our land.*

[F11, aged 23, amputated aged 11]

## Repertory grid findings

As indicated by the mean distances of the various self elements (i.e., self at different times) from the ideal self (see Figure 6.1), the amputees in general viewed themselves as moving away from their ideal selves during the war, and particularly after their amputations. While they had now recovered some degree of self-esteem, it was particularly when playing football that they had a favourable view of themselves, seeing themselves as even closer to their ideal selves than they were before the war. Their view of themselves when playing football seemed to provide a basis for their anticipation of their future selves. These changes in their view of the self at different times are reflected in the relative positions of these different selves in the plot from principal components analysis of the average grid derived from their individual grids (Figure 6.2). Also apparent in this plot is the amputees' very negative view of the perpetrators of their injuries.

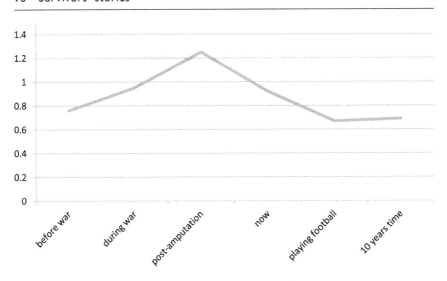

*Figure 6.1*  Distances of self at different times from ideal self

The importance of football in facilitating a more favourable view of the self is also indicated by the fact that the distance of the self when playing football from the ideal self (mean 0.67; standard deviation 0.24) is significantly lower than the distance of the self now (i.e., not specifically when playing football) from the ideal self (mean 0.92; standard deviation 0.28).[8] In addition, as indicated by GRIDSTAT analysis (see Chapter 5), the self when playing football was associated with significantly less conflict (mean 7.90; standard deviation 2.10) than the self now (mean 9.80; standard deviation 2.08).[9] Playing football therefore not only enabled the amputees to view themselves more positively, and even more so than in their rather idyllic memories of life before the war, but also to have a less fragmented and conflicted self-construction.

## Conclusions

The use of forms of extreme violence such as amputation in the civil war in Sierra Leone has been viewed as an attempt to impose humiliation and shame, perhaps as a way of dealing with the perpetrators' own past feelings of humiliation and shame (Keen, 2005). If this is so, the amputees' accounts presented in this chapter indicate that the perpetrators achieved their aim initially, as the experience of shame, as well as guilt and anxiety, is very evident in these accounts. However, also evident in the research findings presented is that it is possible for amputees to recover their self-respect, and that in this particular group of amputees, football played a very significant role in the process of constructing a more favourable, less conflicted view of the self and of the future.

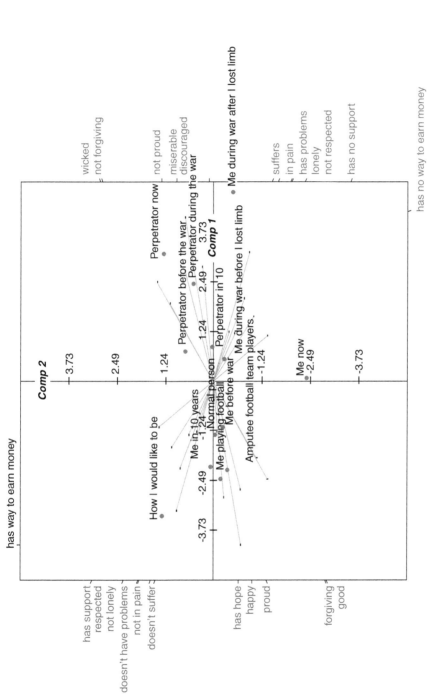

Figure 6.2 Plot of loadings of elements and constructs on first two principal components in average grid of amputee footballers

These resilient and courageous individuals vividly illustrate Kelly's (1955) view, in stating his philosophical position of constructive alternativism, that:

> [T]here are always some alternative constructions to choose among in dealing with the world. No one needs to paint himself into a corner; no one needs to be completely hemmed in by circumstances; no one needs to be the victim of his biography.
>
> (p. 15)

## Notes

1  Further details of the association may be found at www.streetfootballworld.org/network/all-nwm/SHSC or by emailing amputeesoccer@yahoo.com.
2  Some other victims of the rebels were given a choice of the manner of their death, for example whether this was by a bullet, a machete, or burning alive (Human Rights Watch, 1999).
3  This is not dissimilar to current portrayals of beheading as a barbaric Islamic practice, whereas heads have rolled in very many countries and cultures over the years (Larson, 2014).
4  Hands and other body parts were amputated by King Leopold II's brutal regime in the Congo in punishment for villagers failing to fulfil the quotas of rubber that they were expected to collect. As one Belgian official wrote, 'To gather rubber in the district . . . one must cut off hands, noses, and ears' (Hochschild, 2006, p. 165).
5  Twenty-five of these were from the Sierra Leone Single-Leg Amputee Football Club. The other seven were from a group that had broken away from this club in response to an offer of support from an American donor that had failed to materialize.
6  Code numbers of participants are provided in parentheses.
7  Quotes in the third person are from interviews conducted in Krio with the aid of an interpreter.
8  $t = 2.87$; $p < 0.01$; 1-tailed
9  $t = 2.94$; $p < 0.01$; 1-tailed

## References

Hochschild, A. (2006) *King Leopold's ghost: A story of greed, terror and heroism in colonial Africa*. London: Pan.

Human Rights Watch (1999) *Sierra Leone: Getting away with murder, mutilation, rape*. New York: Human Rights Watch.

Keen, D. (2005) *Conflict and collusion in Sierra Leone*. New York: Palgrave.

Kelly, G. A. (1955) *The psychology of personal constructs*. New York: Norton. (Reprinted by Routledge, 1991)

Larson, F. (2014) *Severed: A history of heads lost and heads found*. New York: Liveright.

Manganyi, N. C. (1991) *Treachery and innocence: psychology and racial difference in South Africa*. Johannesburg: Ravan Press.

McCoy, M. (1977) A reconstruction of emotion. In D. Bannister (Ed.), *New perspectives in personal construct theory* (pp. 93–124). London: Academic Press.

Winter, D. A. (2015) Reconstructing life as a one-foot man: Reflections on the role of football. *Journal of Constructivist Psychology*, in press.

Winter, D. A., Wood, N. (2012) *Narrative analysis of loss of limb experiences within a Sierra Leone amputee football team*. Paper presented at 30th International Congress of Psychology, Cape Town.

Yalom, I. D. (1970) *The theory and practice of group psychotherapy*. New York: Basic Books.

# Chapter 7

# Mental health service users' and providers' stories

## Heredity, environment or demons?

The estimated prevalence of mental health problems in Sierra Leone is considerably higher than global rates (currently four times higher for 'severe mental illness' [Alemu et al., 2012]). One reason that has been given for this is the psychological impact of the civil war, and more generally of the violence that has been experienced by 95 per cent of the population in recent years (Asare & Jones, 2005). The legacy of the war, with, for example, the common use of drugs by both child and adult soldiers, includes a very high level of substance abuse. However, as we shall see in Chapter 11, the formal provision of services for mental health problems is very limited, with an estimated 'treatment gap' (the proportion of people with such problems who have not received treatment) of 99.5 per cent. This figure is based on use of formal governmental, non-governmental and faith-based facilities, but excludes more traditional, non-Western services.

In this chapter and the next, we shall present the findings of a series of studies conducted in mental health settings that elucidated the stories of both service users and providers. In this chapter, the focus will be on these individuals' views concerning the causation and treatment of mental health problems; while in the next, the focus will broaden to consider how the interaction between dominant social narratives and individual meaning-making influenced the trajectory of the stories that they told, with particular reference to the civil war.

## Causes and treatment of mental health problems

### Service users' views

The first study sought to elicit the views of service users who were resident in two mental health facilities: Sierra Leone Psychiatric Hospital and the City of Rest, a faith-based rehabilitation centre. The hospital in-patients who participated were six males and two females, with a mean age of 47.13 years (range 27 to 79 years) and lengths of stay ranging from 3 weeks to 27 years. The City of Rest guests (as its residents are termed) who participated were four males and two females, with a mean age of 29.33 years (range 23 to 50 years). All participants were interviewed with a schedule based upon Weiss's (1997) Explanatory Model Interview Catalogue (see Table 7.1).

The interview transcripts were subjected to thematic analysis (Braun and Clarke, 2006), as described by Winter, Bridi, Urbano Giralt & Wood (2011). This indicated various higher-level themes (see Table 7.2), predominant amongst which were practical concerns, relationship issues, and spirituality. Thus, some participants were clear that, in their view, their own problems, or mental health problems in general, were solely caused by a *lack of practical resources*, for example:

*I have no shelter.*

(PH5M, male psychiatric hospital resident, aged 30 years)

*Table 7.1* Interview schedule for service users

1. What do you call the problem which brought you here?
2. What do you think the problem does? Can you tell me more about it?
3. What do you think the natural course of the problem is? What would have happened if you hadn't come here?
4. What do you fear?
5. Why do you think this problem has occurred?
6. How do you think the problem should be treated?
7. How do you want this service to help you?
8. Who do you turn to for help?
9. Who should be involved in decision making about your life?
10. How have these problems affected your life?
11. How would you be without these problems?
12. How effective or helpful has been the help that you have received here on a scale from 1 to 5 (where 5 is highly effective)?
13. What have been the most helpful aspects of the treatment that you have received?
14. What have been the least helpful aspects of the treatment that you have received?
15. What further help do you need?
16. How do you think you will be in a year's time?
17. What do you think are the main causes of mental health problems?
18. What are the best ways of treating mental health problems?
19. How likely are people with mental health problems to recover from those problems?
20. Do you think traditional healing or faith healing can be useful with people with mental health problems?
21. How do you think this approach works?
22. Do you think that drug therapy can be valuable with people with mental health problems?
23. How do you think this approach works?
24. Do you think that counselling or psychotherapy can be valuable with people with mental health problems?
25. How do you think this approach works?
26. What part can their families play in helping people with mental health problems?
27. How can people with mental health problems help themselves to recover?
28. Are there any ways in which mental health services in Sierra Leone can be improved? How could this be achieved?

Table 7.2 Higher-level themes in interview responses

| | |
|---|---|
| Practical/primary concerns | 167 |
| Relationship | 130 |
| Spirituality | 99 |
| Hospital help | 84 |
| Psychological | 71 |
| Deviant behaviour | 69 |
| Traumatic events | 26 |
| Environmental factors | 18 |
| Non-specified treatment | 15 |
| Activities | 15 |
| Education | 14 |
| Proactive behaviour | 11 |
| Calm | 6 |

> *Lack of food, lack of proper homes, no income, no money to put to day to day needs, lack of proper medical care, no clothing.*
> (PH3M, male psychiatric hospital resident, aged 30 years)

Some service users made it clear that the process by which lack of resources led to mental health problems was 'too much thinking', for example:

> *If no money, I think, think, think, my head gets turn.*
> (PH2F, female psychiatric hospital resident, aged 46 years)

> *Frustration, too much thinking – about what if you want something you can't get it.*
> (PH2M, male psychiatric hospital resident, aged 27 years)

Others felt trapped in a vicious circle in which their problems compounded their existing lack of resources. For example:

> *The past two years I have been a downcasted man. I've lost most of my resources, my physical resources, my financial resources, and even my mental resources. The problem has given me severe stress and strain.*
> (PH3M, male psychiatric hospital resident, aged 30 years)

Some service users linked lack of practical resources with *lack of interpersonal resources*. For example:

> *Lack of love, lack of property.*
> (PH6M, male psychiatric hospital resident, aged 79 years)

*The main cause is that I don't have any proper background to continue my studies and there is no proper caring of mother or parents or father for me, there is no proper caring of parents so they make me to become astray without no proper caring.*

(CR4M, male City of Rest resident, aged 24 years)

*Well, I think my parents did not want to take any responsibility. I don't know if they're going according to their procedures about life or what do other people think about us but they don't want to take any responsibility so I think because of that the effect, the effect of seeing other people progressing in life, doing things that is beneficial, I think that they feel annoyed over that. . . .*

(CR5F, female City of Rest resident, aged 23 years)

*When I lost my father and mother. They're both dead.*

(PH3M, male psychiatric hospital resident, aged 30 years)

For several service users, it appeared that any lack of family or social support which contributed to the development of their problems was compounded by the stigma of being diagnosed as mentally ill.

*When you're in hospital, people say you're crazy, don't give you any attention, you're considered a nonentity . . . left in the wilderness. This is how they are, they abandon you but when they hear people are dead they come rushing up to make a big funeral.*

(PH1M, male psychiatric hospital resident, aged 55 years)

*All over the world, not only in Sierra Leone, mental patients are treated as outcasts in society. The families should be encouraged to care for mental patients, giving them the certainty that like malaria or other types of illness the individual will be cured and become an asset to the family.*

(PH6M, male psychiatric hospital resident, aged 79 years)

*. . . it's the encouragement of the parents towards us, that is the main point that cause their discouragement, they're not coming to check on them, they are not sending any clothe for them, they are not visiting them, counsel them frequently, they are not sending any food, they just come and leave us here to the Pastor until the Pastor decide to discharge us so some of us will go. If the Pastor do decide we will stay here until at least 2 or 3 years time.*

(CR5F, female City of Rest resident, aged 23 years)

Another commonly mentioned cause of mental health problems was *drug and alcohol abuse*, for example:

*The main causes of mental problem is that of the taking of drugs like brown brown, cocaine, and so on.*

(CR4M, male City of Rest resident, aged 24 years)

*Because I was drinking – beer, stout, Martell brandy, cognac, Johnny Walker Black Label.*

(PH1M, male psychiatric hospital resident, aged 55 years)

*It's only smoking marijuana cause these mental problems, marijuana. It's marijuana and for Freetown here it's lack of employment, it's lack of employment because the youth are suffering so much that they'll go to college, have their certificate, they'll not be employing, they'll not be employed and some of them don't have trade and so they will go the ghetto and have some marijuana and different types of drugs for them to kill the stress, you see, so that's it.*

(CR1M, male City of Rest resident, aged 30 years)

As indicated in the following quotes, whether practical or psychological issues or drug abuse were emphasized, these were directly related to the *civil war* by some service users.

*Well, I think one cause of mental problems . . . we are just from a war situation and a lot of children were forced to do things that are out of the ordinary like watching people die in front of their faces especially parents, loved ones, friends, they were forced to do things they were not supposed to do like taking drugs, taking part in the massacres, like killing somebody, so the after-effects I think is one of the main problems affecting especially the youths and young adults of this country and secondly depression, stress also leads to the mental problems like if you have no employment or if you have nothing to keep you busy you tend to be idle, you start thinking a lot and especially if it's negative thoughts they tend to build up to a stage where when you get there you can't cope any more.*

(CRM2, male City of Rest resident, aged 26 years)

*Why basically was the war, yes, basically was the war. . . . It was very difficult for me because I had these kids and they were very small and I had to keep moving from one place where I had plans to settle myself because we had plans to settle down in Makene, started building a house there and then we had to run from Makene, we came to Alantown, there again the rebels came and met us and we had to leave all our things, all that we had, collected again beds, pots, pans, and everything that a family needs and we ended up with practically nothing. He [my husband] got so discouraged and he broke down and died and I didn't think that dying was the solution to things. There were still the children to take care of and then, of course the government couldn't afford to employ people . . . and I couldn't get a job. . . . One thing I can say for sure, most of the mental problems experienced in Sierra Leone are due to the war, the desperate type of poverty there is, see, because it's painful if somebody is trying to succeed in life and not being able to make it because of the kind of society you find yourself in, you see there has been a tendency to tribalism, if you're not a member of a particular tribe you don't get into jobs or you don't get promotions in your office, you see, this has been affecting our society adversely, some have even committed suicide because of failure to get scholarships to go overseas, things like that, you see, but with time things might just get better.*

(CRF3, female City of Rest resident, aged 48 years)

For other service users, mental health problems were attributed to *evil spirits*. As one described it:

*It's common with Africans to solicit the help of juju men to hurt those they don't like, those they consider to be their enemy.*

(PH6M, male psychiatric hospital resident, aged 79 years)

Service users' views of life without their problems often seemed to be idealistic fantasies, far removed from their present situations and with little indication of how the vision of a new life could become a reality. For example,

*I would have been OK – with wife and children, perhaps would have money and build a house, have a TV set, video set with games from the Premiership. My team is like Manchester United, Ferguson is coach. When you are here it's just as if you're in a concentration camp.*

(PH1M, male psychiatric hospital resident, aged 55 years)

*Without my problems I would be good, I would be good in the Lord's sight, I would be the happiest man so far in the sight of the Lord and I would try to do the best I could to satisfy my Lord that I am on the earth for a purpose, that I am on the earth for a purpose.*

(CR4M, male City of Rest resident, aged 24 years)

*Well, I think I would be happy at all times . . . making fun with other people, sharing, giving out my own ideas, making fun, having funful things around, you know, reading the Bible, reading novels, going to the cinema, going to the night club, party or show, spending some times in our house drinking and sharing . . .*

(CR5F, female City of Rest resident, aged 23 years)

Consistent with their view of their problems as being due to practical issues, several service users considered that practical help was the appropriate solution to these. Their responses to being asked how their problems would best be treated included the following:

*Need small money so can do business again.*

(PH2F, female psychiatric hospital resident, aged 46 years)

*My problems should be treated by having a place, go back to school and have proper basic necessities, you know, yes.*

(CR4M, male City of Rest resident, aged 24 years)

*Well mostly I think we should try to improve on our environment, try to create jobs, facilities to improve socially on the environment so people especially young adults and youths won't find themselves being idle because the idle mind is the devil's workshop and you find yourself doing things you did not think you'd be capable of doing and you just find yourself that you're stuck on it like glue so one step is for us to have, especially the youths, to have some kind of employment facilities like whatever it is but to just to kill the idleness. Secondly we could improve on the recreational facility let me say sports or other sorts drama or something so people won't find so that the recreations won't tend to be bored and you'll be enjoying yourself at the same time as keeping yourself busy.*

(CR2M, male City of Rest resident, aged 26 years)

In one case the 'treatment' that the service user wanted included, in addition to other practical help, being provided with a woman who would take care of his every need:

*OK, the only solution that problem should have they should give me my own house, marry my woman and giving . . . me a work that I'm doing. I think if I have those things my problem will solve. The woman would take care of me and I would be loved my family, you understand?*

(CR1M, male City of Rest resident, aged 30 years)

Another service user, when asked how his problem should be treated, also emphasized that there should be a combined focus on practical and interpersonal needs:

*Love. I maintain love and money.*

(PH6M, male psychiatric hospital resident, aged 79 years)

In general, service users tended to view the appropriate treatment of mental health problems as being determined by the causation of these. For example:

*If it is a result of cocaine or brown brown or alcohol, the psychiatrist is the most competent. If the mental trouble is the result of a juju man casting a spirit on the individual it is only the juju man who can help the individual and the church can cure the individual by prayer.*

(PH6M, male psychiatric hospital resident, aged 79 years)

*The best way of treating mental problems, you know, everybody have his own problems in different ways and in different categories. Some are demonic problems, some are drug cases. For the drug cases there are certain boys who have aim in life and they have plan for their future career. For the mere fact that they are thinking over those things and they are not having any positive result towards that they take to mind so when they take to mind they go into smoking and drinking alcohol going to different places because there is no progress in their life and they will think that Jesus Christ doesn't care for them and the Almighty God don't care for them knowing that they want the thing to happen for that moment for them to achieve seeing other boys going to Germany, going to America, going to England with big, big cars, having a house, having a wife so they too want to live in that kind of position and achieve that and so they will try to be like those people, they think about that, so they take to mind, you know, so those are the cause for those who are smoking marijuana, you know. . . . The best way of treating mental problems is encouraging the individual 1. in the first place, taking care of all his needs, 2. talking to him, giving him encouraging words, advising him, protecting him, giving him a nice courage and saving him from him not to be going anywhere who the place that you know is a bad place and he will be with you always, and giving him medication, yes and also praying to the almighty God for deliverance and healing.*

(CR1M, male City of Rest resident, aged 30 years)

When questioned about specific types of treatment, service users elaborated on what they considered the active ingredients of these. For example, in relation to drug treatment:

*Makes you sleep and when you wake you're normal.*

(PH1F, female psychiatric hospital resident, aged 55 years)

*Makes you sleep and you forget your problems.*

(PH3M, male psychiatric hospital resident, aged 30 years)

*It removes the toxins from the system.*

(PH6M, male psychiatric hospital resident, aged 79 years)

*They are useful because in the initial analysis the person tends to be excitable and not to sleep so these drugs help the person to sleep, to eat well, and relax so they are useful but the side effects are terrible. There needs to be more research to produce drugs that do not have such terrible side effects, tendencies to convulsions and all those sorts of things.*

(CR3F, male psychiatric hospital resident, aged 48 years)

In relation to counselling and psychotherapy, they tended to view this as a directive, didactic intervention:

*Feel released from the chains of Satan, feel normal.*

(PH1F, female psychiatric hospital resident, aged 55 years)

*If you go by the instructions given to you, that would help you.*

(PH1M, male psychiatric hospital resident, aged 55 years)

*By them encouraging you, talking to you good.*
(PH2M, male psychiatric hospital resident, aged 27 years)

*Yes. It's helpful because by counselling you'll get many ideas for not be going with bad friends by giving you advice, talking to you, giving you good words, words of God, I think those things are good, those things will help you for not to go into temptation, for not to go with, for you not to go to bad places, you will always be with your Bible reading, before going all those odd things. I think your Bible will save you from going into those things.*
(CR1M, male City of Rest resident, aged 30 years)

*Yes, counselling and psychotherapy I believe should be practised more because it's difficult to get into the recesses of human mind, it's not a one-day thing, it's just like a room full of different cupboards and to get into the different cupboards takes time. . . . Well, basically the idea is to give that person confidence in himself or herself, yes, because most of those cases there is a loss of confidence in themselves, not in the world but in themselves.*
(CR3F, female City of Rest resident, aged 48 years)

Most service users also saw a potential role for faith healing and/or traditional healing, although they tended to be more ambivalent about the help of juju men:

*Faith healing works through the help of God by delivering you from the mental problem. Traditional healing through the help of skilled herbalist gives you proper build up of your body.*
(PH3M, male psychiatric hospital resident, aged 30 years)

*Well, with faith healing the guest is taught to believe that God is there with him in his problems and that with constant prayer solutions will come to his problems or her problems and, you see, that gives the victim an inner sense of peace because whether you like it or not stress plays a great role in the malfunctioning of anybody's mind.*
(CR3F, female City of Rest resident, aged 48 years)

*Through by believing in Christ Jesus and believing in his Father and you know that you are the child of God and you must stay focused with God, and he or she must stay focused with God. [Does traditional healing help at all?] Well, for me in my own belief I think sometimes traditional beliefs it works in those that believe in it but as for me I do not believe so I believe in Jesus and his Father and I think they do my healing for me.*
(CR4M, male City of Rest resident, aged 24 years)

*You pray to the Lord Almighty, have faith in God, ask him to . . . recover; or go to the Juju man, medicine man, some of them tell you lies, tell you this medicine does so but it is not the correct thing.*
(PH1M, male psychiatric hospital resident, aged 55 years)

Several service users were appreciative of the treatment that they had received. For example:

> *We bless the nurses all the time. They are mothers and fathers, encourage us, bath us, give us clothes, and food, come and do therapy with us, we bless them, plait our hair.*
>
> (PH1F, female psychiatric hospital resident, aged 55 years)

> *The hospital has helped me greatly because they've given me the love I lacked. Sometimes they give me 5 or 6 cola nuts and when I start to chew it I become happy. Nurse Y gives me covering for the cold at night, which I don't get from my relatives. They want me to be an eyesore in society. It's due to the help that I received from some of the nurses – not all though.*
>
> (PH6M, male psychiatric hospital resident, aged 79 years)

> *This place have helped me a lot because they have made me to know Jesus, my saviour and lord and they have made me pray always and I have had my deliverance so I thank God for that, that the place have made me well through the Lord Jesus.*
>
> (CR4M, male City of Rest resident, aged 24 years)

One psychiatric hospital resident found the following aspects of treatment helpful:

> *At times when you're sick, when you go off[1], they give you Largactil. At times they put you in the cell. At times you're chained to the bed. Largactil injection – tranquillizer for the brain. The matron helps us, used to dash us[2], give us money, at times. Gives us medicine at times when we're ill.*
>
> (PH1M, male psychiatric hospital resident, aged 55 years)

However, he found it unhelpful:

> *when they don't look after you at all when you become aggressive.*

Others were very critical of their care, or perceived lack of this, for example:

> *the way the nurses treat the patients is not good. Nurses are partial, they will do good to one patient but to another one they will not do anything. . . . Give me Largactil to sleep, tablet for cold in foot[3] . . . I have no other treatment. There is no helpful here. . . . They got grudge to me because I ran away last time so when they brought me now they chained me to stay indoors. . . .*
>
> (PH4M, male psychiatric hospital resident, aged 55 years)

> *Not sufficient food, no light, we are not earning money, and I have no job. I want a job.*
>
> (PH5M, male psychiatric hospital resident, aged 30 years)

A passive, fatalistic outlook, and dependence on God, was evident in many of the service users. Thus, asked what had caused his problems, one service user replied:

*Only God knows, I don't know.*
(PH2M, male psychiatric hospital resident, aged 27 years)

Asked how they saw their future, a common response was:

*It's left to God.*
(PH2F, female psychiatric hospital resident, aged 46 years)

Similarly, asked how she thought that her problem should be treated, one service user responded:

*It's left with you, anything you want to do.*
(PH1F, female psychiatric hospital resident, aged 55 years)

A similar passivity was also often evident when interviewees were asked how service users might help themselves to recover. For example:

*You shouldn't ask that question. When you say mental patient, he's senseless, he doesn't know good from bad, how will he be able to help himself unless people help him?*
(PH6M, male psychiatric hospital resident, aged 79 years)

*Well, people with mental problems I don't think if they can help themself, they'll be just going backward except there is someone that is clever amongst them that will be able to treat them, to give them first aid, and take them to pastors for deliverance and prayer.*
(CR4M, male City of Rest resident, aged 23 years)

## Service providers' views

Interviews were also conducted with a senior staff member in Sierra Leone Psychiatric Hospital, two pastors at the City of Rest, and the president of the National Union of Traditional Healers.

The psychiatric hospital staff member presented a holistic view of the causation and treatment of mental health problems:

*Ah, yes, some of the causes of mental health problems . . . are economical, social, of course psychological, of course due to peer pressure experimentation for young patients although of course people have this misconception that I won't fail to add that they are caused by other things but scientifically I would not want to mention that because they are caused by demons, whatever, some people think that but it's a misconception, yes, yes. Socio-economical, psychological, of course lastly and honestly I may not know, which is idiopathic, I may not know, so whatever you do science will not even try to find out that so it's very difficult for you, that goes beyond one's imagination. So basically those are the ones, socioeconomic, experimentation, peer pressure, yes, yes.*

In regard to treatment:

*Well, best ways could be twofold, maybe as an inpatient or outpatient, then of course medications, occupational therapy, psychotherapy, of course counselling, and then letting the patients engage in some life activities that may help them after discharge. There are so many, multifacets, you attack them from so many angles, a holistic approach to the patients.*

This approach included an acknowledgement of the value of traditional healing for people who believed in this:

*Well, because people who seek this help have a more than 50 or 60 per cent belief already in this healing, I think that is what helps them to cope with whatever the traditional healer will tell them because while going there they already believe that these people might help me and you get help from what you believe in so that's what I want to say. If you believe you take this thing and it will work then it's going to work. If you believe it cannot work even if you take a drum of it it cannot work. So the people already have that mindset that traditional healing helps them so them going there is another step forward to their healing process. . . . Honestly, most of the people that might benefit are the people who live in the provinces and then, of course, less educated people. Few of them will come for orthodox or psychological treatment.*

The City of Rest pastors distinguished between problems with demonic and non-demonic causes, and, as indicated in Table 7.3, one of them was able to differentiate the characteristics of people with these two types of problems. While the pastors viewed both types of problem as amenable to faith healing, they considered that only non-demonic problems could be helped by Western medicine and that if a demonic problem were treated by traditional healing, this could make the problem worse:

*Well, traditional healing of course, but maybe that cannot be a permanent cure because people who have gone through traditional healing for mental sickness, sooner or later they're attacked back again and become more worse. The Bible says when somebody's demon possessed and that demon is cast out the demon will go and find somewhere it will pay a visit to the temple and sooner or later . . . it will be free, that demon will go and hire other wicked demons and they will come and the end result is that person will become more worse than before, but when they're treated spiritually when the demon is cast out there is no reason for them to return back.*

*Table 7.3* City of Rest pastor's view of characteristics of people with demonic and non-demonic problems

| Demonic | Non-Demonic |
| --- | --- |
| **(demon of murder, demon of suicide, etc.)** | **(most drug problems; pressure-related problems)** |
| become violent | think wisely |
| use abusive language | think positively |
| keep self untidy | behave normally and decently |
| look at one place for long | talk sensible |
| fight and sometimes kill | love people |
| can injure self | organized |
| sometimes deny food; others eat a lot | gentle |
| sometimes do not sleep | forgive |
| sometimes keep themselves filthy | conscious of good and evil |
| | when get temptation, try to resist |
| | when asked to pray, they do it |

The president of the National Union of Traditional Healers had a more elaborate taxonomy of 'different types of madness':

> *The first one that makes people to go into madness is frustration. That one can make you to go into madness because you don't have a helper, somebody who can help you, that one can make you go crazy. The other one we have germs within our brain, we have within the skull there, that one can make you to go mad. . . . The third one that makes people go crazy . . . sometimes the native people they use a herbal way to make you go crazy, because of jealousy. The fourth one, some people have a devil, they can see like I'm talking to you now, because they have not fulfilled an agreement with the devil they make you to be mad. . . . There are 5 types of crazy. Some people they go to take treatment. They don't go to the right doctor, they go to a different type of doctor. Some are using syringes that are used for veterinary purposes, they are used to inject people. They are not qualified and they use syringe to inject people, they make people go off. . . . Another thing that make you go crazy is that some people are taking drugs, cocaine, that will make you to go off.*

He indicated that he was able to treat each of these types of madness with different herbs, in addition to his skills in curing other illnesses, including HIV infection, and in carrying out operations without cutting the patient. To demonstrate his prowess, and to encourage financial support for the opening of a hospital for traditional healing, he was taking people with long-standing mental health problems off the streets and attempting to show that he could cure them. Indeed, the interviewer (David) was then taken to see one of these people, a half-naked young woman who was kept in chains in a yard behind the traditional healer's office.

In his view, Western medicine was ineffective with many such people (except drug abusers), as it was not rooted in Sierra Leone culture:

> *When somebody has gone crazed, maybe he has some devil or djinn that makes him to go off, maybe he has some medicine that has disturbed the brain, those who knows the witchcraft will be able to detect and cure witch people. You are not part of the society, you will not be able to cure them. That is why we, the union, can cure such people because we know the society and we know what is happening. You the medical doctor can cure all the disease that is natural given to somebody or brought to somebody through God so that is why a lot of medical doctors will not be able to cure people.*

### Student health workers' views

Views concerning the causation and treatment of mental health problems were also explored in two groups of students. One group consisted of 20 male and 10 female fourth-year medical students (mean age 25.17 years; range 22 to 34 years) who were receiving their first set of lectures on psychiatry and clinical psychology. The other consisted of 33 male and 14 female community health officers (mean age 31.85 years; range 22 to 49 years) attending teaching sessions on mental health problems.

The method used in these studies was repertory grid technique (see Chapter 5). With the medical students, at the first of their lectures they were asked to list types of mental health problems, and then to agree which were the 12 most common of these. The final list, which constituted the 'elements' in the grid, consisted of *dementia, schizophrenia, manic depression, seizures, phobic disorders, drug abuse, multiple personality disorder, psychosis, hysteria, post-traumatic stress disorder, depression* and *obsessions.* Fourteen construct poles (descriptors) were supplied, based largely upon possible causes and methods of treatment of mental health problems which had been mentioned either in discussion with the class concerning these topics or in the interviews conducted with service users and providers. These were *hereditary, caused by infection, caused by spirit possession, caused by stress, caused by problems in family or marriage, caused by lack of faith, caused by poverty, dangerous, curable, can be helped by medicine, can be helped by a juju man, can be helped by faith healing, can be helped by counselling or psychotherapy and benefits from practical help (e.g., money, job).* Participants were asked to rate each of the elements on a 7-point scale on each construct (where 7 indicated that the element was very much described by the characteristic listed above and 1 that it was very much not described by the characteristic) at their first lecture and again at their last lecture, eight days later. Due to an oversight, a construct pole of *can be helped by a traditional healer* was omitted from the first grid, but this was included in the second grid.

Individual grids were analyzed by the Idiogrid software (Grice, 2002), which also allowed the derivation and analysis of an average grid of the group at each assessment session and a differential changes grid comparing these two average grids. The statistical method of principal components analysis, when applied to the average grid from the first assessment, indicated that the medical students' major dimension of construing mental health problems (reflected in the first principal component) contrasted hereditary problems, and those caused by infection, which could be helped by medicine, with those caused by difficulties in the family or marriage, stress or poverty, and which could benefit from practical help or counselling and psychotherapy. Seizures and dementia were construed in the former terms, and contrasted with depression, drug abuse and post-traumatic stress disorder. The first principal component of the post-teaching grid was essentially similar to that in the first grid.

The students' second most important way of construing mental health problems (reflected in the second principal component) contrasted problems caused by spirit possession with those which could be helped by medicine, and which are dangerous. It contrasted phobic disorder and obsessions with seizures. In the second principal component of the post-treatment grid, the contrast to problems which could be helped by medicine was problems which could be helped by counselling and psychotherapy.

In the pre-teaching average grid, correlations between constructs provided further indications that students' views concerning the appropriate treatment of particular mental health problems were determined by how they believed these problems to be caused (see Table 7.4). In the post-teaching grid, constructs referring to ways of helping differentiated less between elements, and this was particularly so for the constructs concerning practical help and faith healing. Comparison of the mean ratings on constructs in the pre- and post-teaching grids indicated a significant decrease in the extent to which problems were seen as being caused by spirit possession[4] and a significant increase in the extent to which they were seen as hereditary[5] or caused by marital and family problems,[6] curable,[7] and able to be helped by medicine.[8] However, the correlation of 0.88 between the two average grids indicated that overall there had been little change in the students' construing of mental health problems over the course of lectures.

Correlations between individual grids and the average grid were moderately high, indicating commonality in the students' views, apart from the grid of one student, whose construing deviated markedly from the consensus of the group at both assessments. Examination of his grid indicated that, unlike most of the other students, he firmly believed that various mental health problems, including dementia, schizophrenia, phobias, drug abuse, depression, and seizures, were caused by spirit possession, and apart from reconstruing of phobias this view changed very little during teaching.

*Table 7.4* Problems appropriately and inappropriately treated by different approaches as indicated by correlations between constructs in the medical students' average pre-teaching grid

| Type of treatment | Appropriate problem | Inappropriate problem |
| --- | --- | --- |
| medicine | caused by infection<br>dangerous | caused by lack of faith |
| counselling/psychotherapy | marital/family problems<br>caused by stress<br>caused by lack of faith<br>caused by poverty | caused by infection<br>hereditary |
| juju man | caused by spirit possession | |
| faith healing | caused by poverty<br>caused by lack of faith<br>marital/family problems<br>caused by stress<br>curable | |
| practical help | caused by poverty<br>caused by lack of faith<br>marital/family problems<br>caused by stress<br>curable | |

A similar procedure was used with the group of student community health officers. They viewed the 12 most common mental health problems, which were then used as the elements in a grid, as *drug-induced psychosis, epilepsy, post-traumatic stress disorder, depression, obsessive compulsive disorder, puerperal psychosis, schizophrenia, senile dementia, phobia, meningitis, anxiety,* and *mania.* The 12 construct poles on which they rated these problems were possible causes of mental health problems provided by the class, together with ways of dealing with them. They were as follows: *caused by frustration or loss, caused by trauma or stress, caused by abuse, caused by infection, caused by problems in childhood, caused by a biochemical disorder, caused by social and economic factors, caused by curses or demonic possession, can be helped by medication, can be helped by a juju man, can be helped by counselling or psychotherapy and can be helped by a traditional healer.*

Principal components analysis of the average grid of this group indicated that their major way of construing mental health problems (reflected in the first principal component) contrasted those caused by infection, which could be helped by medicine, with those caused by frustration or loss, which could be helped by counselling or psychotherapy. Meningitis, epilepsy, and puerperal psychosis were construed in the former terms, and depression and drug-induced psychosis in the latter. As with the medical students, correlations between constructs indicated that student community health officers' views concerning the appropriate treatment of particular problems were determined by their views concerning the problems' causation (see Table 7.5).

*Table 7.5* Problems appropriately and inappropriately treated by different approaches as indicated by correlations between constructs in the student community health officers' average pre-teaching grid

| Type of treatment | Appropriate problem | Inappropriate problem |
|---|---|---|
| medicine | caused by infection<br>caused by childhood problems<br>biochemical | |
| counselling/<br>psychotherapy | caused by frustration/loss<br>caused by abuse<br>caused by socioeconomic factors | caused by infection |
| juju man | caused by curses/demonic possession | |
| traditional healing | caused by curses/demonic possession<br>biochemical | |

## Chaining

These investigations of service users', providers', and students' construing indicate generally differentiated construing of mental health problems, in which a range of Western and more traditional treatment options are considered, depending upon the perceived causation of the problems. However, as we shall discuss further in Chapter 11, the choices available to people presenting with such problems in Sierra Leone tend to be much more stark. As indicated in some of the service users' accounts, they include a high probability of being kept in chains.

Since staff members' reasons for chaining psychiatric hospital in-patients were often unclear, these were explored using personal construct methods. One method used was an adaptation of ABC technique (Tschudi, 1977; Tschudi & Winter, 2010), in which the senior staff members on four wards were individually given the construct 'chained – unchained' and were asked to give positive implications of being unchained and negative implications of being chained; and, conversely, negative implications of being unchained and positive implications of being chained. Table 7.6 presents a composite of the responses of three staff members, of whose patients two-thirds were chained, and who expressed similar views. They regarded the disadvantages of chaining as including physical problems and deterioration of personal hygiene, but the advantages as including restriction of access to illicit drugs and of opportunities to cause trouble and harm. Although none of the seven in-patients on the fourth staff member's ward were currently chained, she was unable to think of a single disadvantage of chaining, the perceived advantages of which for her were preventing aggression, the person's own protection, and ensuring that medication is administered.

Five senior staff members also completed a repertory grid in which four chained and four unchained in-patients on each of their wards were rated on 22 construct poles (descriptors). The latter were largely based upon the previous studies but also included constructs concerning the feelings elicited in staff by the in-patients. They were as follows: *mentally ill; possessed by demons; addicted to drugs or alcohol; under stress; has problems due to the war; has problems in family or marriage; has few resources (money, home, or job); dangerous; curable; bad/wicked; sad; can be helped by drugs; can be helped by counselling or psychotherapy; can be helped by occupational therapy; can be helped by juju man; can be helped by faith healing and prayer; can be helped by traditional healer; should be in chains; makes me feel afraid; person I can talk to; like me in character; and thinks too much.*

Principal components analysis of the average grid of four of the staff members (one grid was excluded as it was incomplete) showed a clear distinction of the chained from the unchained patients on the first principal component, which differentiated patients who should be in chains, could be helped by occupational therapy, and are dangerous from those who are curable and mentally ill. This can be seen in Figure 7.1, which provides a plot of loadings of elements and constructs on the first (represented by the horizontal axis) and second (represented by the vertical axis) principal components, and in which the chained patients, on the right of the plot, are separated from the unchained patients, on the left.

Since mental illness therefore did not seem to be the basis for the decision to chain particular individuals, what *was* this decision based upon? Some clues are provided by the repertory grid. For example, it can be seen that patients who should be chained were viewed as being like the staff members in character. Drawing upon Landfield's (1954) exemplification hypothesis of threat, could it be that staff were threatened by those patients who reminded them

*Table 7.6* Responses of three staff members (D, P, J) to 'chaining' ABC

| (Participants were asked to indicate the positive and negative implications of each pole of construct a1-a2; constructs b1-b2 indicate the disadvantages of a1 and advantages of a2; constructs c1-c2 indicate the advantages of a1 and disadvantages of a2.) | |
|---|---|
| a1  chained | a2  unchained |
| b1  causes oedema of feet (J) | b2  no oedema |
| restricted freedom of movement (J) | can use toilet |
| (urinate where they sit) | |
| personal hygiene deteriorates (J) | personal hygiene preserved |
| get foot drop (D) | no foot drop |
| freedom ceases/restricts movement (P) | able to move about/go to toilet |
| c2  restrained from moving around (J) | c1  access to drugs |
| won't harm each other (J) | harm each other |
| don't cause trouble (J) | cause trouble |
| can give them medication (D) | they go out |
| don't take drugs (D) | abscond to take drugs |
| calm state (under control) until effect of drugs (J) | leave hospital/cause problem outside (be aggressive; attack people; harmful) |

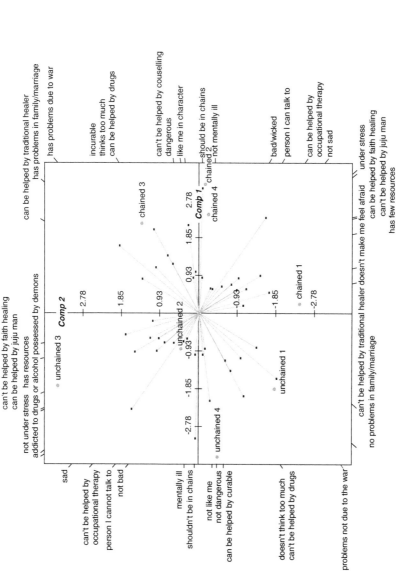

*Figure 7.1* Plot of elements in construct space from principal components analysis of average grid concerning staff members' construing of chained and unchained in-patients.

of some aspect of themselves that they had rejected but could all too easily revert to, and that chaining served to reinforce the distinction between staff members and these patients? A further clue is provided by the finding that the average percentage sum of squares (a measure of how extremely they were construed) accounted for by the chained patients was significantly lower than that accounted for by the unchained patients.[9] This perhaps indicates that the chained patients were less construable, and therefore more anxiety provoking, to staff than were the unchained patients. It suggests that when staff found patients hard to understand, they dealt with the anxiety that this caused by keeping the patients in chains.

The preferred option for these staff members may, in any case, have been not to try to understand their patients. In the words of a Koranko proverb, 'When a mad man speaks, a mad man understands him' (Hinzen, James, Sorie & Tamu, 1987, p. 198). The implication is that it is not possible to understand a mad man, and not worth trying to do so, unless one is mad oneself, and furthermore that it would be threatening to find that one did have some glimpse of understanding of the mad man's view of the world because one would then have to question one's own sanity. Far better, then, to keep the mad man in chains and to adopt a purely custodial approach which does not necessitate attempts at understanding.

## Conclusions

The high reported prevalence of mental health problems in Sierra Leone can be ascribed to the civil war and its aftermath. While clearly the war was not directly a factor in the mental health problems of everyone diagnosed with these, many of the stories of residents in the psychiatric hospital and the City of Rest implicated the war and subsequent lack of practical and interpersonal resources, or substance abuse which again was often a legacy of the war. Both service users and staff acknowledged a variety of causes of mental health problems, and correspondingly of different possible treatment approaches. However, treatment options are very limited and largely custodial, including the chaining of residents in mental health facilities, perhaps as a way of dealing with the anxiety and threat which these individuals elicit in staff.

## Notes

1   'Go off', 'go to mind', and 'go crazed' are expressions for becoming disturbed.
2   'Dash' means to give some money to.
3   As a result of being chained.
4   $t = 2.15$; $p < 0.05$
5   $t = 3.09$; $p = 0.005$
6   $t = 2.12$; $p < 0.05$
7   $t = 2.59$; $p < 0.05$
8   $t = 3.29$; $p < 0.01$
9   sign test: $x = 0$; 1-tailed $p < 0.05$

# References

Alemu, W., Funk, M., Gakurah, T., Bash-Taqi, D., Bruni, A., Sinclair, J., Kobie, A., Muana, A., Samai, M., Eaton J. (2012) *WHO profile on mental health in development (WHO proMIND): Sierra Leone.* Geneva: World Health Organization.

Asare, J., Jones, L. (2005) Tackling mental health in Sierra Leone. *British Medical Journal,* 331(7519): 720.

Braun, V., Clarke, V. (2006) Using thematic analysis in psychology. *Qualitative Research in Psychology,* 3: 77–101.

Grice, J. W. (2002) Idiogrid: Software for the management and analysis of repertory grids. *Behavioral Research Methods, Instruments, & Computers,* 34: 338–341.

Hinzen, H., James, F. B., Sorie, J. M., Tamu, A. T. (1987) *Fishing in rivers of Sierra Leone: Oral literature.* Freetown: People's Educational Association of Sierra Leone.

Landfield, A. W. (1954) A movement interpretation of threat. *Journal of Abnormal and Social Psychology,* 49: 529–532.

Tschudi, F. (1977) Loaded and honest questions: A construct theory view of symptoms and therapy. In D. Bannister (Ed.), *New perspectives in personal construct psychology* (pp. 321–350). London: Academic Press.

Tschudi, F., Winter, D. (2010) The ABC model revisited. In P. Caputi, L. L. Viney, B. M. Walker, N. Crittenden (Eds.), *Personal construct methodology* (pp. 89–108). Chichester: Wiley-Blackwell.

Weiss, M. (1997) Explanatory model interview catalogue (EMIC): Framework for comparative study of illness. *Transcultural Psychiatry,* 34: 235–263.

Winter, D., Bridi, S., Urbano Giralt, S., Wood, N. (2011) Loosening the chains of preemptive construing: Constructions of psychological disorder and its treatment in Sierra Leone. In D. Stojnov, V. Džanovic, J. Pavlovi, M. Frances (Eds.), *Personal construct psychology in an accelerating world* (pp. 95–108). Belgrade: Serbian Constructivist Association/EPCA Publications.

# Chapter 8

# Stories from within mental health settings

## Social context as a frame and a chain

Chapter 7 focused on mental health service users' and providers' views concerning the causation and treatment of mental health problems in Sierra Leone. This chapter now broadens this discussion through presenting *stories from within mental health settings* that consider how service users and providers responded following the civil war in Sierra Leone. The discussion considers how the interaction *between* dominant social narratives and individual meaning-making influenced the trajectory of stories people were able to tell and therefore their relative experiences of distress.

As highlighted in Chapters 2 and 10, the focus on one response trajectory regarding how people react following trauma (post-traumatic stress disorder, or PTSD) within the current literature base has been criticized for being too narrow. Concern stems from the privileging of Western understandings of the self, negating to consider sufficiently the role of context; that is, the available social, cultural and political discourses. This has potentially led to the development of models and theories which could be considered culturally insensitive, if applied outside of the context from which they have derived.

According to Smedslund (1984), culture constitutes the 'invisible obvious' in psychology. Indeed, Voestermans (1992) describes the seeming failure to consider how mental processes may be affected by culture as the Achilles heel of psychological research. These points are further explored in Chapters 11 and 14. An example of research (Brown, 2013) which was conducted in Sierra Leone and brings the relevance of culture to the foreground of understanding individuals' and communities' responses following trauma is now presented.

### Research question

How does social context influence how people respond over time following trauma?

### Method

#### Participants

As shown in Table 8.1, ten service users and staff from two 'mental health' organizations in Sierra Leone were interviewed. There were eight individual

Table 8.1 Demographics of participants

| Participant | Position | Age | Gender | Religion |
|---|---|---|---|---|
| Isatu | Staff | 58 | Male | Christian |
| Selina | Staff | 53 | Female | Christian |
| Nasratha | Service User | 40 | Female | Christian |
| Abdou | Staff | 44 | Male | Muslim |
| Group (Ishmael, Sadiu, Gabriel) | Service Users | 34, 44, 57 | 3x Male | Undisclosed |
| Tamba | Staff | 42 | Male | Muslim/Christian |
| Fodey | Service User | 42 | Male | Muslim |
| Gladi | Staff | 48 | Female | Christian |
| Gabriel | Service User | 34 | Male | Christian |

interviews and one group interview; one of the individual participants was also a group member.

The only exclusion criterion was for individuals who were currently experiencing significant distress or who were likely to experience a negative impact on their well-being if they took part in the interview. The central inclusion criterion was that participants appraised themselves as having experienced significant distress during the war, alongside the ability to communicate in English.

## Interview method

The epistemological stance taken throughout this research was social constructionism. This position holds that there is no ultimate truth to be 'discovered' through research, only the socially and personally constructed truths of individuals. These truths are constructed through relationships with others and through the discourses available to us within our past, current and future imagined social environment.

Manganyi (1991) argues that life-story interviewing is a suitable methodology within the African context, focusing as it does on the 'creation of meaning, after an approximate actuality and a truth supposed possible brought about by systematic witnessing . . .' (p. 75).

Thus, the qualitative research methodology of narrative analysis was chosen. This approach offers the opportunity to consider the influence of broader cultural narratives upon individual stories. Moreover, rather than focusing on specific events, narrative analysis can consider the development of story telling across time (Wells, 2011), therefore offering researchers the opportunity to position identity as co-constructed, changeable and contextual.

Semi-structured individual interviews were then carried out. The interview schedule is outlined in Table 8.2. All participants had experienced the civil war. It was felt that analyzing the stories of people who are presumed to be currently

*Table 8.2* Interview schedule

*Group interview:*

1. Could you tell me about what you, as a community, have been through since the end of the Civil War?
   - What has helped people to keep going?
   - What are the strengths within your community?
   - What has been difficult for your community since the war?
2. What was life like for your community before the war?
   - Do you notice any changes in your community?
   - What is different now?
3. What do you think the future will be like for your community?
   - What do you hope for?

*Individual interviews:*

1. Would you be able to tell me about what life was like for you before the Civil War?
   - What was life like when you were a child?
2. Could you tell me about what you, personally, have been through since the end of the Civil War?
   - What has life been like?
3. Have there been things that have helped you to keep going?
4. Where do you draw your strength from?
5. What has been hard for you along the way?
   - How did you get through the hard times? What helped?
6. Do you think you have changed as a person?
   - In what way?
7. Compared to others around you has your story been similar or different?
   - What aspects are similar/different?
8. What are your hopes for the future?

in distress ('service users') together with those experiencing less distress (the staff members) would potentially allow different response trajectories to be heard and considered. Further, the rationale for interviewing both individuals and a group lay in the idea that cultural or 'master' narratives are created and transmitted 'between' people. Therefore, it was hypothesized that the collection of group accounts would provide a valuable microcosm for analyzing how stories are told in a public setting as compared to the more private setting of an individual interview.

## Procedure of transcription and analysis

The interviews were transcribed with all utterances from both the interviewee and the researcher included. Given the language barrier, extended effort was made to transcribe the interviews as accurately as possible. Consultation was sought with a Sierra Leonean colleague who held specialist knowledge of the local dialect and culture. Reflexivity is the realization that researchers are part of the social world that they study (Frank, 2012). Thus, a reflective diary was used as a tool to increase the credibility and rigour of the research and was viewed as essential information for the analysis regarding the impact of the researchers' assumptions from their own differing cultural context.

An 'experience-centred' approach (Andrews, Squire & Tamboukou, 2013) was taken throughout the analysis with a focus on the contextual, dialogic and performance elements of the narratives. Each interview was listened to numerous times with the transcript. Notes were first made on the narrative content of the stories. This was achieved by highlighting the different relative points in the participant's narrative throughout the transcript. For example, the beginning, middle and end points of the overarching narrative were highlighted alongside the smaller storylines within the bigger narrative. This content was not 'coded' but instead summarized for each individual participant and across the participants.

Once a sense of the emerging storylines within the interview had been achieved and summarized, the interviews were listened to with a focus on the organization, performative, and dialogic elements of the narrative. As Riessman (2003) highlights, the researcher does not find narratives but instead participates in their creation. An important part of the context of a story is the person to whom the story is being told.

The next stage of the analysis focused on which 'master' or 'dominant' narratives stood out across the interviews (Bamberg, 2004). The concept of master narratives refers to the 'big stories' available in the context, for example regarding how one should cope following war. At this stage, information from the reflective diary and anthropological and fictional material relevant to the context (e.g., Conteh, 2011; Ferme, 2001; Shaw, 2009) was also considered. Once the researchers had developed some initial ideas about the master narratives which seemed to inform and frame the stories, the interview accounts were reread with these hypothesized 'master narratives' in mind. The final stage of the analysis involved a focus on what was implicit or only alluded to within the narratives. This process involved reviewing the notes from the individual analysis with a focus on what was mentioned but not elaborated. The questions in Table 8.3 provided a framework for this analysis.

*Table 8.3* The guiding framework for analysis

a) What are the main themes (storylines), 'the feel of life', and the narrative arc (across time)?
b) What does the way the story was told say about meaning (for the narrator, for the researchers)?
c) For whom was this story constructed and for what purpose?
d) How has context (social, political, cultural discourses) influenced what has been said (or not said)?
e) What cultural resources does the story draw on/take for granted?
f) How have I (as a researcher) influenced what has been said?
g) During turn taking, which stories are advanced and how?
h) Are there gaps and inconsistencies which might suggest preferred, alternative or counter narratives?

## Results

The results of this study indicated that context, the dominant social discourses, both framed and 'chained' personal response. Importantly, there was not a significant narrative difference observed between the stories told by service users and service providers. Two master narratives stood out through the analysis: first, *Because of Almighty God, We Forgive*, and, second, *Bear It, and Forget*. Results suggested that these dominant social discourses may have also silenced and therefore 'chained' certain storylines. Examples of the influence of each master narrative upon the individual and collective stories will be presented, follow by illustrations of the storylines which may have remained constrained. However, first the results of the group interview will be briefly discussed.

As Bamberg (2004) highlights, countering master narratives is not necessarily an easy accomplishment. This struggle was demonstrated within the group interviews where one of the participants put across strongly the story 'Because of Almighty God, We Forgive',

> It's all about faith. We try to control our mind. Right? Allow God to speak in our mind like 'don't revenge. Leave this individual for me to judge' this individual.
>
> (Gabriel, group interview)

When another of the group members (Ishmael) asked the question, '*Do you think the war is ended?*', Gabriel reaffirmed the dominant view – his view – that the war is over. Then instead of following up what Ishmael was trying to question, the interview moved on. Ishmael's story that '*the war is not over*', that all is not forgotten, was silenced and remained untold. This is an example of a dynamic that was observed across the group interview.

The interaction between the dominant and counter narratives within the group interview can perhaps provide a glimpse at how difficult it was to hold onto a different viewpoint other than '*Because of Almighty God, We Forgive*'. This highlights in praxis how context may have shaped the performance of participants' stories. Whilst limited, this dynamic may also provide some insight into how the war was talked about, or not talked about, in everyday 'public' conversation, therefore indicating the social process through which individual stories may become framed and constrained.

### Because of almighty God, we forgive: How were the stories framed by this dominant discourse?

The presence of God and forgiveness within the individual narratives was significant. All but one of the tellers used the character of God as a conduit for making sense of their experiences and decision to forgive and move on.

> We allow God to speak in our mind to forgive, that's why we are living as a community now.
>
> (Gabriel, group interview)

For some, God was spoken of as a main character throughout the narrative, whereas for other people, religion was only utilized as a meaning-making tool, perhaps when there was no other way to make sense of their lives. In this way, for some, God was storied as the ultimate 'saviour', whereas for others he was positioned as a 'source of strength' – to make a *self-determined* change. Alternatively, a number of accounts utilized both of these resources within their narratives.

> *Well, I must say, after the war, first of all, I rehabilitated myself I see that the only hope I have is God, the almighty God, you see, and I pray to him so that he can give me strength to begin*

> (Abdou)

Here, the theme of religion and God as the only hope, an unfailing belief, falls *alongside* the idea of personal rehabilitation.

### How were the stories 'chained' by this dominant discourse?

There was only one interviewee who did not use God as a significant character in the narrative, either as a saviour or as a strength. In this narrative God was only referenced in relation to basic survival, as a force which could decide whether someone lived or died but not as a tool to make sense of what had happened. The plotlines of God as a saviour or as a source of strength are the most 'visible' and clear storylines across the narratives. However, some participants also alluded to a sense of doubt about whether their faith could fully explain the horror and pain they experienced, or the challenges in society which remained. This doubt was mainly expressed through the way stories were told, the performance, rather than the content of what was said. However, in some of the stories the participants did explicitly question 'Why, God?'. This explicit storyline was most prominent in one participant's narrative. Throughout his narrative, he questioned why the war happened when he and his people had '*not done anything to nobody*'.

> *We don't know what we doing, nothing we no do to nobody (hmmm) but the rebel come, anybody they want do bad to they do to, do bad to.*

> (Isatu)

### Bear it, and forget: How were the stories framed by this discourse?

> *All of us are managing. . . . It's something in your community. It means you're also strong. When you're strong, you will do something. Well, we are managing.*

> (Selina)

The focus across the narratives was on survival and the meeting of practical needs, on 'bearing it', rather than perhaps the emotional journey or intrapsychic process. Across the narratives there did not seem to be an overt sense of an individual emotional struggle to make sense of experiences. The dominant collective story seemed to suggest that if you could 'bear it' and 'forget', this would enable you to move on and survive. A simple, yet striking, physical description of coping was used,

> You just sit down.
>
> (Selina)

However, results also indicated that there was a tension across the stories regarding whether one 'bears it' as an individual or as a community. Across the narratives a struggle stood out where some participants attempted to negotiate the integration of the historically dominant culture discourse that 'we bear it' alongside the new individual experience that 'everyone is on their own'. For some people the nature of the war meant that they were left to cope alone, to 'creep on their own knee' (Gabriel).

> Everyone is on his own. Doing things. Everyone by herself or himself, or his family anyway. So I just have to say so . . . because everyone is doing good although things are hard . . .
>
> (Selina)

### How were the stories 'chained' by this dominant discourse?

Analysis of the performative aspects of the accounts suggested that it may have been more challenging for participants to forgive and forget than what was first revealed within the content.

> Some forget, some don't forget.
>
> (Isatu)

Some accounts were told in a way that suggests that the teller was almost reliving the experience through the retelling. A pattern across the narratives seemed to unfold where people would start to tell a 'coherent' faith-based story, 'Because of Almighty God, We Forgive', but revert to a more chaotic account, before returning to conclude that it was thanks to God that everything is now okay.

> So we just listen to fiery fiery fiery (hmmm) all over the Katbaton they come to Wellington, Kissy so many fiery (hmmm) in that night. So I have a small children with me boys, (Okay) my daughter yeah. . . . So I so torment that time, so I just open the door I peep in the house I (ummm) I see so many people . . . come in the city (hmmm) . . . because this just past now we everybody try to forget about war problem (hmmm) now we pray God, new something come having us life Sierra Leone now so encourage me then we forget everything. . . .
>
> (Isatu)

In fact, one participant's story had very few moments of 'coherence'; although he did not explicitly use the words 'I cannot forgive or forget', the way the story was told allows the listener to glimpse the difficulty involved in forgetting. Frank (1995) conceptualizes this type of story, or non-story, as a 'chaos' story and high-lights that it may be viewed as a heroic attempt to portray 'reality', rather than adopt the master narrative.

The way that the two master narratives may have influenced what was said and not said within the narrative accounts has been presented. These results will now be discussed with reference to the implications and relevance for theory and everyday clinical practice.

## Discussion

The aim of this research study was to explore how social context influences personal response following trauma. The results have indicated that the context, the available social, cultural and political discourses in society, both framed and 'chained' personal response.

### Understanding the influence of context

From a social constructionist position, knowledge is constructed between people, through language (Burr, 2003). Narratives are not just ways of seeing the world, but we actively construct the world through the stories we tell and the stories we hear (Murray, 2003). The primary resources for telling a new story are the stories that are already circulating in the setting (Frank, 2012). This research highlighted two main dominant discourses as the primary cultural resources which framed and constrained the stories of personal and collective responses told within interview. So, what evidence is there to support the existence of the identified dominant discourses?

### Because of almighty God, we forgive

Unlike conceptions of God in the West, in Sierra Leone God is 'the ultimate source of all power' (Sawyer, 1970, as cited in Conteh, 2011). God is considered the ultimate cause of a person's fortune or misfortune in life and death, with the ultimate responsibility for everything. In Sierra Leone God is highly visible everywhere, and religious leaders played a large part in the peace agenda.

As described by Conteh (2011), 'Wherever the African is he/she is with his/her religion' (p. 85). Post-colonial civil wars in Africa, like previous civil wars and anti-colonial resistance, have been known to have strong religious elements (Conteh, 2011). After the war in Sierra Leone, religious leaders preached far and wide the message of forgiveness (Shaw, 2009). However, it is also noted that in public discourses religion is portrayed solely as influencing reconciliation. In 1997, the Inter-Religious Council of Sierra Leone (IRCSL) set the objective to equip and mobilize cooperation efforts among religious communities (Conteh, 2011). Further, the council took concrete steps towards restoring stability, reconciliation and renewal (Kganu, 2001, as cited in Conteh, 2011). The IRCSL succeeded not only in bringing together the head of state, rebel leaders, and all those who had a part in the conflict, but was also able to persuade the warring factions to agree to talk and find a peaceful resolution (Conteh, 2011). In 2000 the IRCSL created a working proposal, to be implemented by both Muslims and Christians, for reconstruction and renewal in Sierra Leone. This included a national campaign for confession, forgiveness, reconciliation and renewal. As Conteh (2011) highlights, Article 7(2) of the Truth and Reconciliation Act refers to the assistance from traditional and religious leaders in facilitating reconciliation. Religion played a major part in establishing peace in Sierra Leone. Following the war the message '*Because of Almighty God, Forgive*' was loud, powerful and clear.

### Bear it, and forget

In Sierra Leonean culture, pain is seen as an unavoidable part of life, and a person is expected to bear it (Jackson, 2004). Sierra Leoneans are pragmatists, and a focus on one's own inner feelings and thoughts is far less pronounced in Africa than in the West (Jackson, 2004).

Instead, the focus is on survival and the meeting of practical needs. Shaw (2009) talks about how different regions and localities have their own memory practices and their own techniques of social recovery, developed during the course of their own history. Most people in Sierra Leone prefer the 'forgive and forget' approach to 'truth and reconciliation' rather than the Western model of 'revealing is healing' (Shaw, 2009). The preference for social recovery through a 'forgive and forget' strategy rather than a 'talk' strategy can be understood in a context where fear of retaliation and government reprisal is ever present. In Sierra Leone social forgetting is seen as the refusal to reproduce violence by talking about it publicly (Shaw, 2009). The message '*Bear It, and Forget*' historically draws from stories within the context about how best to manage adversity, implying that if one can bear it there is more chance of being able to move on and survive another day.

### Stories 'chained'

Foucault (1982) states that the cultural context of a story will dictate what can be said and what is 'illegitimate'. Power structures which try to represent a 'truth' can become oppressive, and it is critically important to consider the stories that fall outside of, or remain constrained and 'chained' by, the dominant discourses. As Bamberg (2004) notes,

> If it is possible to delineate more clearly where and how discourses that run counter to hegemonic discourses emerge, and if it is possible to describe the

fabric of these counter discourses we should be able to make headway in designing alternative strategies to public, institutionalised power relations.

(p. 353)

Whilst the less dominant storyline 'Why, God?' was present in some of the stories, it was not explicitly mentioned in all the narratives. Perhaps in the context of Sierra Leone, where religion is interlinked with society, explicit questioning of this discourse could lead to further social rejection. Questioning God may be seen to be associated with, or permitted by, 'madness'. In this way, the social context may influence personal response by silencing some stories.

In considering the complexity of language and communication, Coordinated Management of Meaning (CMM; Pearce, 1999) contrasts *unknown stories*, which are not currently possible to tell, with *untold stories*, which the participants are capable of telling but have chosen not to. *Unheard stories* are then those which, although they have been told, have not been heard, perhaps because they are in conflict with dominant discourses. CMM suggests that a spiralling process may unfold, where unheard stories become untold stories, and untold stories become, after a while, unknown stories (Pearce, 1999). Foucault (1982) talked about how the complex power relationships in every aspect of our social, cultural and political lives can lead us to internalize the norms and values that prevail within the social order. Therefore, some discourses remain 'illegitimate' or silenced; some stories remain unintegrated and in chaos. Perhaps these are the people who then attract the label of 'mentally ill'. These ideas are further discussed in Chapter 14, where the impact of political and societal inequality upon distress, what we call mental illness, is considered by exploring the influence of power in relation to the biomedical model and Global Mental Health Agenda (GMHA).

### Trajectories

The described research (Brown, 2013) indicates that the interaction between context and individual construing influences the trajectory of the story told, the *type* of response which is observed. Participants who told the more dominant cultural story (that 'We Bear It' or 'Because of Almighty God') seemed to embody more of a restitutive (Frank, 1995) or recovery trajectory across their narrative. That is, their narratives depicted difficulty from which they ultimately recovered, and so the direction of travel within their story stayed the same. In Western culture such people may be described as 'resilient'. Research shows that in situations of adversity, resilience is observed when individuals engage in behaviours that help them to navigate their way to the resources they need to flourish (Ungar, 2013). However, the personal agency of individuals to navigate and negotiate what they need is dependent upon the capacity and willingness of people's social ecologies to meet those needs (Ungar, 2013); for example, the flexibility of a society to consider and hear alternative stories and ways of construing events.

Within the research, those participants who demonstrated a 'struggle' with the tension of conflicting beliefs or cultural ideas (for example, God as saviour vs. strength), perhaps because their immediate social environment allowed them the flexibility to do this, seemed to demonstrate within their narratives an integration between past and new beliefs. The 'feel' of the story took on more of a 'growth' trajectory. This means that the plot of the story encompassed the identification of difficulty of which they initially struggled to make sense, but which ultimately resulted in them making a change which went beyond their previous functioning into a preferred direction. These types of narrative fit with what has most commonly been conceptualized in the Western world as 'post-traumatic growth'.

Alternatively, what stood out across the narratives was that the narratives of individuals who struggled to make personal sense of their experience via the dominant social discourses (for example, 'Because of Almighty God') seemed to remain in 'chaos' (Frank, 1995). Chaos stories are non-stories which typically do not include a resolution. To translate this finding into the language most commonly used in Western psychological literature, people who tell chaos stories are likely to fit descriptions of a 'traumatized' person, as someone who may fit the diagnostic criteria for PTSD, compound or complex trauma, that is, someone who is struggling to make sense of and, thereby, meaningfully story and process their experience.

Considering a social ecological interpretation of resilience, Ungar (2013) emphasizes how a resource is only useful if it is valued. The discourse 'Because of Almighty God, We Forgive' is only useful if it makes sense to the individual. Individual resilience occurs when there is an environment that facilitates access to resources and willingness from those who control resources to provide what individuals need in ways that are congruent with their culture (Ungar, 2013). Thus, there is a relational context involved in how people respond following trauma which encompasses the fit between the prominent discourses within a community and an individual's personal sense making.

When individuals and communities experience ongoing trauma and adversity such as civil war, they understandably search for a way to story and make sense out of their experience. Straker (2013) refers to this experience as continuous traumatic stress (CTS), which is observably different to the one-off event-focused trauma which PTSD in Western culture is often associated with. As in the case of Sierra Leone, a society may attempt to provide master narratives to support communities' recovery; however, such cultural discourses may not be accessible for all or may be heard to greater or lesser degrees depending on the individual or the cultural context. This research suggests that for individuals and communities to 'recover' and 'grow' following trauma, the environment, the social ecology, needs to be able to support, hear and honour different stories. People need to be supported and encouraged to tolerate multiple truths; God can be the ultimate saviour, a source of strength, and a decision-making force. Some aspects of survival can be negotiated as a community, and some struggles must be traversed alone.

In this conceptualization the social context is seen as highly influential in the development and perpetuation of distress, growth and resilience. Through this research (Brown, 2013) we can clearly see the relevance that social context plays in how people cope and manage following trauma. The implications of this research are discussed in Part 3: Implications.

## Conclusions

If we are to move forward in our knowledge regarding the psychological impact of trauma, then we must make a commitment to valuing the influence of context in our academic writing, theories, models and clinical practice. As Bamberg (2004) noted, complicity and countering go hand in hand. Now is the time to step back and critically question how we can support people's attempt to resist dominant discourses, rather than label them as unwell or traumatized.

## References

Andrews, M., Squire, C., Tamboukou, M. (Eds.) (2013) *Doing narrative research*. London: Sage.

Bamberg, M. (2004) Considering counter narratives. In M. Bamberg, M. Andrews (Eds.), *Considering counter narratives: Narrating, resisting, making sense* (pp. 351–371). Amsterdam: John Benjamins.

Brown, R. (2013) *'I Fall Down, I Get Up': Stories of survival and resistance following civil war in Sierra Leone*. Unpublished doctoral thesis. University of Hertfordshire, United Kingdom.

Burr, V. (2003) *Social constructionism*. London: Routledge.

Conteh, S. (2011) *Major religions of Sierra Leone*. Canada: Xlibris.

Ferme, C. M. (2001) *The underneath of things: Violence, history, and the everyday in Sierra Leone*. Oakland: University of California Press.

Foucault, M. (1982) The subject and power. *Critical Inquiry, 8*(4): 777–795.

Frank, A. W. (1995) *The wounded storyteller: Body, illness, and ethics*. Chicago: University of Chicago Press.

Frank, A. W. (2012) Practicing dialogical narrative analysis. In J. A. Holstein, J. F. Gubrium (Eds.), *Varieties of narrative analysis* (pp. 33–52). London: Sage.

Jackson, M. (2004) *In Sierra Leone*. Durham, NC, & London: Duke University Press Books.

Manganyi, N. C. (1991) *Treachery and innocence: Psychology and racial difference in South Africa*. Johannesburg: Ravan Press.

Murray, M. (2003) Narrative psychology. In J. Smith (Ed.), *Qualitative psychology: A practical guide to research methods*. London: Sage.

Pearce, W. B. (1999) *The coordinated management of meaning*. A Pearce Associates seminar. Available at: http://www.pearceassociates.com/essays/cmm_seminar.pdf [Accessed 15 May 2013].

Riessman, C. K. (2003) Analysis of personal narratives. In J. A. Holstein, J. F. Gubrium (Eds.), *Inside interviewing: New lenses, new concerns* (pp. 331–347). London: Sage.

Shaw, R. (2009) *Rethinking truth and reconciliation commissions: Lessons from Sierra Leone*. Washington, DC: United States Institute of Peace.

Smedslund, J. (1984) The invisible obvious: Culture in psychology. In K. Lagerspetz, P. Niemi (Eds.), *Psychology in the 1990s* (pp. 443–452). Amsterdam: North-Holland.

Straker, G. (2013) Continuous traumatic stress: Personal reflections 25 years on. *Peace and Conflict: Journal of Peace Psychology,* 19(2): 209.

Ungar, M. (2013) Resilience, trauma, context, and culture. *Trauma, Violence, & Abuse,* 14(3): 255–266.

Voestermans, P. (1992) Psychological practice as a cultural phenomenon. *New Ideas in Psychology,* 10: 331–346.

Wells, K. (2011) *Narrative inquiry.* Oxford: Oxford University Press.

# Chapter 9

# Refugees' stories
## Walking for your life

> *While every refugee's story is different and their anguish personal, they all share a common thread of uncommon courage – the courage not only to survive, but to persevere and rebuild their shattered lives.*
>
> Antonio Guterres, United Nations High Commissioner for Refugees (June 2005; paragraph 2)

Population displacement is accelerating across the world at a rapid rate (United Nations High Commissioner for Refugees, 1975–2011), and forced migration remains one of the most devastating effects of civil war. Forced migration is defined as that which has an element of coercion to it, including perceived threats to life. Despite more than 200 studies investigating the plight of forced migrants and refugees (Fazel, Wheeler & Danesh, 2005; Hollifield et al., 2002), research has been limited to predominantly large-scale, quantitative analyses of psychiatric symptoms (Ryan, Dooley & Benson, 2008) or the impact of environmental factors, such as economic security (Moore & Shellman, 2006). We present here a qualitative study of a non-clinical population. It provides a holistic view of the refugee experience, including greater insight into the decision to take flight, followed by subsequent experiences in the host country. According to Adhikari (2012, p. 590), 'Why some people choose to stay while others choose to leave continues to be an interesting and important subject of inquiry'. We also examine refugees' attitudes to those responsible for war atrocities and their ability to forgive.

When considering the plight of refugees fleeing war zones, it would be reasonable to assume that this is purely to escape physical danger. However, Adhikari (2012) argues that conflict alone is not the sole factor affecting people's decisions to leave. He proposes a choice rationale, in which individuals make the decision to leave or stay based on a diverse range of secondary factors, including economic and social vulnerability. Others have identified additional secondary factors, including Moore and Shellman (2006), who demonstrated that political terror is associated with higher levels of forced migration. Furthermore, Melander and Oberg (2007) reported that the geographical spread of a conflict, rather than its brutality, is a greater predictor of fleeing from a conflict zone. Kelly (1955), however, would suggest that the decision will be the alternative which the individual can most accurately predict.

## Theories of migrant well-being

Displaced from their place of origin, migrants are obliged to adapt to a new environment, and theories have been devised by several authors to describe post-migration adaptation. These include the medical model, psychosocial stress models, the acculturation framework, and conservation of resources models. As mentioned earlier, the overwhelming focus has been on mental health (Fazel et al., 2005), consistent with the medical model. Whilst an understanding of trauma is essential in considering the plight of refugees, the medical model exaggerates the link between pre-migratory trauma and the image of refugee populations as predominantly 'sick' (Carlson & Rosser-Hogan, 1991). It focuses on high-impact events that occurred pre-migration, thereby completely overlooking any resettlement issues. Consequently, its ability to assess migrant adaptation processes and the impact of host country environment on psychological well-being is limited.

Conversely, sociocultural models are primarily concerned with the demands of interacting effectively in a new environment (Ward & Kennedy, 1999). Lazarus and Folkman (1984) approached this in terms of demand versus resources. In their model, emphasis is placed on cultural coping strategies facilitated by psychological, social, and economic resources. This model possesses an advantage over the medical model in that it does not pathologize psychological distress; rather, it conceptualizes it as a normal response to major life changes in the absence of adequate resources. This 'resource stress' model also forms the foundations of Berry's (1997) 'acculturation framework', which goes further by specifically incorporating cross-cultural transitions. There are two major issues: the extent to which the individual is involved with his or her original 'heritage' culture and the 'dominant' host culture. Despite its descriptive and explanatory power (Ouarasse & Vijver, 2005), it could be suggested that intercultural demands are exaggerated in this model, thereby minimizing the difficulties originating from elsewhere in the migratory experience. This criticism is particularly relevant where refugees have moved to a neighbouring country, similar to their own, which is in fact the case for the majority of the world's 15.4 million refugees (United Nations High Commissioner for Refugees, 2013).

Silove and Franz (1997), Hobfoll (1998, 2001) and Ryan, Dooley and Benson (2008) propose models of migrant well-being based on the conservation of resources (COR). COR theory sees the key component of any psychological distress as a result of resource loss, which is unavoidable in forced migration. It suggests that extreme trauma undermines various adaptive mechanisms (Silove &

Franz, 1997). With adequate resources, these mechanisms can be restored, but where resources are unavailable, psychological stress is inevitable.

Whilst describing aspects of migration, these models could be accused of failing to describe the entire forced migratory experience. Personal construct psychology, however, could provide an alternative and more detailed perspective.

## Constructivist approach

The guiding theory to this study of refugees is personal construct psychology (PCP) (Kelly, 1955) (see Chapter 2). The principal assumption is that individuals continuously devise, test, and revise personal theories to help make sense of the world and anticipate future experiences (Hardison & Neimeyer, 2012). Kelly (1955) describes how constructs that originally appeared workable can later be invalidated by new events, such as those involved in migration. As detailed by Winter (1992, p. 16), 'Optimally, construing and its transitions proceed in cyclical fashion, and involve a flexible response to new experiences, whether these be validating or invalidating, including a balanced use of strategies in response to invalidation'. This is particularly pertinent to the plight of refugees, who will be required to construe and reconstrue following the many novel events involved in their forced migratory experiences. If refugees possess constructs determined in their place of origin that are unable to admit the novel elements presented in their new environment, this presents difficulties both in adaptation and general mental well-being. If adaptation is unsuccessful, the person may experience depression and a sense of alienation. Alienation is a significant issue facing refugees. Kelly (1969) stated that to retain personal autonomy, external power is sacrificed, with the resultant powerlessness a form of alienation (Winter, Patient & Sundin, 2009). Combined with Foucault's (1980) suggestion that an individual can only validate his or her constructs if they are consistent with the dominant discourse, there are obvious causes for alienation in refugees who, upon arrival into a new culture, are at the whim of an alien culture's thoughts and processes. This can be compounded by a further sense of powerlessness in being unable to anticipate what the future holds, this being determined by the bureaucracy of the host country rather than by the individual. Alienation resulting from cultural estrangement and social isolation is also pertinent to refugees. In the former, individuals find themselves unable to reconcile their own construing with that of their social group. In social isolation, the individual may choose to withdraw from society in order to find safe refuge to validate their own construing, or is isolated by others who find it difficult to understand their constructs and subsequently find them unpredictable.

The significance of the individual's social and cultural context is noted in PCP (Butt, 1996, 2000; Davidson & Reser, 1996; Epting, Prichard, Leitner & Dunnet, 1996; Kelly, 1955; Procter, 2016; Scheer, 2000). People belonging to the same cultural group may construe and anticipate events in the same way, creating personal meanings that are bound to the influence of their society and the historical, economic and political environment. The construction of culture, providing this framework of meaning, can be said to mediate all relationships (Leitner, Begley & Faidley, 1996), and hence its importance should not be underestimated. Indeed, Oliver and Schlutsmeyer (2006) suggest that the construct system that we develop is assembled by and in our interactions with others, and we silently absorb aspects of our cultural environment. This is particularly salient to displaced populations who have been settled in culturally different surroundings. Those who proceed to cultural integration have been able to construe the new culture extensively and accurately and make appropriate changes in their construct system. Burr, Giliberto and Butt (2013) suggest that a more successful reconstruing process takes place when the preexisting construct system is sufficiently permeable to incorporate constructs when in a new situation. However, as Scheer (2003) points out, when living in a new environment, the potential for invalidation of the individual's construing is greater. Correspondingly, the ability to predict accurately what others will do and adjust one's own behaviour accordingly (Kelly, 1963) is important in forced migration, as refugees are required to adapt to a new culture and its behaviours.

Many factors interact in the individual's decision to migrate. Kelly (1955) states that given a choice, individuals select the alternative that they anticipate will best enable them to predict their worlds. That is, their choice will allow either for the validation of their current construct system or for an acceptable extension to it, rather than it being based on maximizing pleasure (Kelly, 1995). This is the 'Choice Corollary'. In the area of forced migration, individuals possess minimal information regarding the alternatives available to them. Consequently, they will have heightened difficulty in predicting an outcome, thus adding to the complexity of the decision process and the impact on their construing.

### The Experience Cycle

To function optimally, an individual's construing and its transitions proceed in a cyclical fashion. If a prediction is validated, the construct system is likely to be preserved, but if invalidated, the construct system is more likely to be modified. Kelly (1970) elaborates this in the Experience Cycle (Figure 9.1). It involves the anticipation of an event, the individual's investment in this anticipation, encounter with the event, dis/confirmation of the anticipation and revision of the person's construing if necessary.

Research on refugees from a PCP perspective is somewhat limited. An exception is Sermpezis and Winter's (2010) study of asylum seekers. This describes re-traumatization on arrival in the host nation and suggests a state of liminality, in which the host nation fails to engage the asylum seeker group. This chapter includes further examination of these ideas.

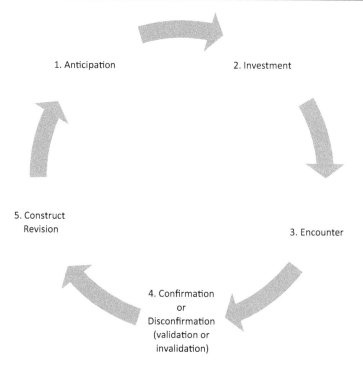

1. Anticipation

2. Investment

5. Construct
   Revision

3. Encounter

4. Confirmation
   or
   Disconfirmation
   (validation or
   invalidation)

*Figure 9.1*   The Experience Cycle (Oades & Patterson, 2016). From Oades, L. G., Patterson, F. (2016) Experience Cycle Methodology: a qualitative method to understand the process of revising personal constructs. In D. A. Winter, N. Reed (eds.). *Wiley handbook of personal construct psychology*. Chichester; Wiley-Blackwell. Reproduced by permission of John Wiley & Sons Ltd.

## Forced migration from Sierra Leone

As discussed in Chapter 4, Sierra Leone experienced heightened forced migration during the period of its civil war (1991–2002). The war was characterized by extremely high levels of violence and frequent shifting of allegiances (Wood, 2008). An estimated 50,000 were killed and over 1 million displaced (Human Rights Watch, 1999). Elements of the army were colluding with rebels throughout the war (Bellows & Miguel, 2006), and as a result the main victims of violence were civilians rather than combatants. Violence was indiscriminate and fear of imminent death was endemic in the population (Keen, 2005). A dramatic increase was observed in net migration figures from the country during the civil war (Figure 9.2). Outside of the African continent, the United Kingdom is the most popular host destination for Sierra Leonean migrants. There were 22,898 Sierra Leonean citizens resident in the United Kingdom in 2012 (International Organisation for Migration [IOM], 2015). Seventeen thousand Sierra Leonean migrants arrived in the United Kingdom during the period

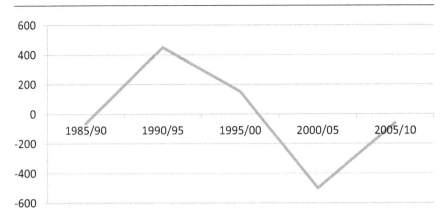

*Figure 9.2* Net migration from Sierra Leone 1985–2010 (total number of emigrants less total number of immigrants per year in thousands: a negative number indicates net immigration). Derived from data provided by United Nations, Department for Economic and Social Affairs, Population Division, Population Estimates and Projections Section (United Nations, 2015)

of the war (Rutter, 2003), which equates to approximately 75 per cent of the present total, and included the loss to Sierra Leone of an estimated 30 per cent of its highly educated nationals (Stevens, 2012), depriving the country of much of the skilled workforce required to address ongoing poverty and underdevelopment. The impact of forced migration on individuals and source and host states is substantial. With conflicts continually erupting throughout the world and forced migration increasing, an approach which takes a holistic view of the forced migratory experience is an important and useful method of research. Information on individuals' construing both before and after migration will help enlighten understanding and policy making. In addition, investigation of migrants' construing of those responsible for war atrocities and their forgiveness will assist in post-conflict reconstruction.

The study reported in this chapter aimed to describe the participants' Experience Cycles on moving to the United Kingdom. Of particular interest to the study were forgiveness and resilience (Goins, Winter, Sundin, Patient & Aslan, 2012), and whether time had any impact on these. These were included due to their inherent importance in the psychological well-being of individuals and the reconciliation of communities.

## Research methods

Six participants aged between 39 and 73 years took part in the study: four female, two male. All were resident in Sierra Leone for part or all of the civil war. Although participants' religious beliefs were not requested, all six volunteered this information. Four (female) participants were Muslim (we named them Farah, Karimah, Mouna, and Shazia), and two (males) were Christian (Thomas and Simon).

As mentioned in Chapter 6, an interview method was considered the most appropriate due to the rich history of oral story telling in Sierra Leone. Each participant was asked questions based on those outlined in Table 9.1, derived from Experience Cycle Methodology (Oades & Viney, 2000), and their responses were recorded in digital format.

The interview attempted to elucidate an understanding of the construing of participants' past, present and future; their Experience Cycle in migrating; and how they construe/d those responsible for war atrocities. The narratives were coded into Experience Cycle phase categories (Table 9.2), in order to examine

*Table 9.1* Interview schedule with Sierra Leonean migrants

*I would like to hear your life story including your experience of the war in Sierra Leone and your experiences of living in the UK.*

*What are the main factors you considered when you were thinking about leaving Sierra Leone?*

*What were your main concerns? (Were you concerned about physical danger?)*

*What options did you see open to yourself at this time?*

*What predictions and expectations did you have of life in the UK?*

*How much did you want these predictions to come true? How much did it matter to you at the time?*

*How has life been in the UK compared to how you thought it would be?*

*How do you feel about this?*

*What have you learnt from this experience?*

*Has your experience of moving to the UK changed the way you view things or how you behave?*

*If it happened again, would you do anything differently as a result of your experience? (What things would you change?)*

*Would you see different options open to you now if it happened again?*

*How well do you think the government is doing at achieving a peaceful state? (restorative justice, political/institutional systems, acknowledgement of suffering)*

*How well do you think the citizens of Sierra Leone are adapting to life after the war? (understanding of the reasons for the war, understanding of the psychological and social pressures on perpetrators, ability to forgive perpetrators, remorse as a requirement for forgiveness)*

*Would you describe yourself as highly work orientated? (leader? values family and friend relationships? high achiever?)*

*Do you feel able to forgive those responsible for the war atrocities in Sierra Leone?*

*Table 9.2* Category groupings of Experience Cycle Methodology data

| Phase | Group | |
| --- | --- | --- |
| Anticipation | (1) Tight prediction | (2) Loose prediction |
| Investment | (1) High investment | (2) Low investment |
| (Dis)confirmation | (1) Validation | (2) Invalidation |
| Construct revision | (1) Significant revision | (2) Minimal revision |

the 'construct change pathway' (Oades & Viney, 2000, 2012). In addition, any major themes emerging from the participants' experiences were identified through thematic content analysis (TCA) (Braun & Clarke, 2006).

Finally, refugee perceptions were also examined using repertory grid technique (see Chapter 5). The elements were: *me in the UK now; me in Sierra Leone before the war; me in Sierra Leone during the war; me when I first arrived in the UK; me in 10 years time; a Sierra Leone resident in Sierra Leone now; how I would like to be; the individuals responsible for war atrocities now; the individuals responsible for war atrocities before the war; the individuals responsible for war atrocities during the war; the individuals responsible for war atrocities in 10 years time; asylum seekers in the UK now; a British citizen now.* Ten constructs were elicited from each participant using Kelly's (1955) triadic method. In addition, two constructs were supplied by the researcher: *resilient – not resilient* and *forgiving – not forgiving.* Participants provided a rating on a 7-point scale for each element on each construct, the preferred pole receiving a score of 7.

## Findings

We found that all six participants' narrative descriptions were consistent with Kelly's (1955) Experience Cycle. None revised their construal as a result of the experience of moving to the United Kingdom. A commonly held tight prediction of 'safe sanctuary' was validated in all cases. Analysis of repertory grids demonstrated changes in construal of the self and war perpetrators over time. For all participants, the largest divergence from ideal self was observed during the war. Two participants, Thomas and Karimah, showed the most variation in construal with regards to forgiveness and resilience across different time points. For others, the ability to forgive was lost after the war began and violent atrocities had been experienced. Thematic analysis of participants' narratives revealed four common, overarching themes. These were (1) the need to escape to safety; (2) the changing experience of life in Sierra Leone; (3) individual determination; and (4) forgiveness.

### Participants' Experience Cycles

It had been expected that life in the United Kingdom would have been anticipated by each participant using a unique and complex set of constructions and that a degree of reconstruing would have occurred where anticipations were not met. On the contrary, all six participants displayed extremely similar Experience Cycles. Each held a tight and superordinate prediction that the United Kingdom would provide a safe refuge. This was supported by results from repertory grid analyses and thematic analysis, both emphasizing an overriding concern with safety. As one participant, Mouna, describes:

> . . . *they shoot my friend next to me, they shoot boom, the bullet caught her, she was dead and I was thinking tomorrow, maybe that's my time . . . so I had to get out [to the United Kingdom].*

All the participants considered themselves highly invested in their move to the United Kingdom, which predominantly involved the abandoning of loved ones and, for some, the loss of financial and social status. Some variation between participants was observed in the encounter phase of the Experience Cycle. Here, narratives diverged in detailed accounts of departure from Sierra Leone and arrival in the United Kingdom. Half of the participants, Farah, Karimah and Shazia, arrived to known contacts whilst the remainder, Thomas, Mouna and Simon, arrived alone, requiring them to establish themselves without initial support. Despite these differences, all six found that their expectation of the United Kingdom as a safe sanctuary was confirmed and no construct revision was required. In fact, the construct of the United Kingdom as a sanctuary was continuing to be 'crystallized' (Sewell, 2005), as it continued to prove itself a safe location and because participants continued to endow physical safety with great importance. This was possibly due to the enduring impact of the heinous events they experienced during the war. Confronted with the likelihood of death, participants acted to preserve their construct system by physically removing themselves from the situation. As Ryan, Dooley and Benson (2008) contend, the basic psychological need of living in a safe environment has increased psychological significance for those fleeing conflict. With core structures at stake, it is unsurprising that safety was of preeminent importance. To be able to anticipate a future in an alien country and avoid associated anxiety, the individual's construct system requires an ordinal structure in which superordinate constructs provide predictions that can be validated and are permeable to novel events. A superordinate construct concerning 'safety' appeared to subsume many other constructs. Thus, subsequent to extreme physical threat, numerous construct-invalidating events can be tolerated (subsumed) provided that the individual's physical integrity remains intact.

> *They want to kill me . . . that's why I run away . . . and we are walking with no food for 20 days, no washing . . . you are walking for your life.*
>
> (Karimah)

In the initial stages of conflict, society members will form beliefs (constructs) that provide a meaningful picture, reduce uncertainty, and allow them to make predictions about the future (Bar-Tal, 2000). Given the notorious uncertainty of conflict zones, it could be suggested that participants were pushed beyond this initial construct formation and were required to choose between the alternatives of certain safety in the United Kingdom versus the uncertainty of death or violent attack in Sierra Leone. Migrating to the United Kingdom would provide the alternative that could be most readily validated. This was also evident in one of the major themes emerging from thematic analysis, that life in Sierra Leone was a changing experience, with associated uncertainty. Adhikari (2012, p. 594) found that refugees' choice of destination state is 'a function of their relative expectations of being victimized'. Alternatively, with limited information regarding life in the United Kingdom, participants may have worked through their construct hierarchy and based their choice on a superordinate factor they could predict: safety.

> *. . . when the war came everything was just, everything goes. I don't know what to say, it was not like before . . . so you come here [to the United Kingdom, because] it's much better, much safer.*

(Shazia)

In the process of forced migration, refugees are compelled to experience many new and unfamiliar events. In order to negotiate their way successfully, they need to develop constructs that can adequately admit elements outside their original range of convenience (the elements to which they are usually applied) and accommodate various and inevitable invalidations resulting from new experiences. The evidently flourishing lives of the participants in this study indicated that their construct systems had successfully evolved to adapt to their new lives in the United Kingdom. More detailed exploration of participants' experiences would be interesting and may reveal whether all of the participants' constructs were equally permeable in the sense of being able to be applied to new events and experiences. It is possible that participants may retain some constructs from their place of origin, and these may remain impermeable to novel events in the United Kingdom. In such cases the individual would be unable to reconstrue in response to invalidation.

An additional explanation for the participants' success in adapting to British life is an ability to predict another's behaviour through knowledge and understanding of others' construal processes. This has increased complexity in a foreign country where cultural norms and nuances will affect construing. The participants in our study appear to have become successfully accustomed to the construing of the UK population.

> *I enjoy living here. I like London, I like the people.*

(Simon)

Of particular interest in this study was the fact that all six participants' Experience Cycles indicated the superordinacy of safety. Whilst individual construct systems are unique, people from the same cultural background tend to construe certain events in a similar way, that is, they may develop certain constructs within the same historical, political or cultural context. As Murray-Prior (1998, p. 549) explains, 'It is not assumed that individuals develop similar construct systems because they have the same experiences, only that, because of their various experiences, they have come to the same hypotheses about the results of various actions.' According to Bar-Tal (2000), in extended conflicts, personal constructs become societal constructs and contribute greatly to a society's identity. This may have been the case in our study sample, where the shared experience of conflict insecurity resulted in all of the participants construing the alternatives available to them, including the United Kingdom, in terms of safety.

### Participants' construing of self and war perpetrators

Our repertory grid analyses looking at the percentage sum of squares for elements (a measure of the salience of each element for the individual) indicated that the relative importance of self and war perpetrators varied between participants and across time points (before and during the war; on arrival to the United Kingdom; now; and in 10 years). For Farah and Mouna, war perpetrators were more salient than self whether before, during, or after the war. For Thomas, Karimah and Simon, the time point of 'during the war' held most saliency. For Shazia, post-war time points were most prominent. Without more detailed investigation, it is difficult to explain the reasons behind the variations between individual participants. However, it is highly likely that individual differences and distinct, unique conflict experiences have had an effect.

As indicated by the mean distance of the various elements from the ideal self, participants displayed most closeness to their ideal self (indicating high self-esteem) now, in 10 years, and before the war. They all perceived that the greatest difference between self and ideal self was during the war. This may be due to a shifting from their core roles and associated guilt during the conflict. War perpetrators were construed as the most dissimilar to ideal self for all participants. However, variation across time was observed: Farah and Thomas construed war perpetrators as most dissimilar during the war, as might well be expected. More surprisingly, the remaining participants construed war perpetrators now as the most dissimilar. As repertory grids may access a person's construing at a lower level of awareness, it may be that the chronological importance of 'now' was most prominent to participants. Alternatively, participants may have been unable to accept 'war perpetrators now' into the range of their constructs. Thus, despite the likelihood of change since the war, participants were unable to reconstrue war perpetrators. On the other hand, a superordinate construction, such as 'blame', may have subsumed the more detailed constructs that may well have demonstrated changes over time.

Of interest was the participants' construing of asylum seekers and British citizens. Farah, Karimah, and Simon construed a British citizen as closer to their ideal, suggesting an aspiration to being like the British. Florczyk (2014) found that those immigrants who showed positive attitudes towards British culture tended to report more positive feelings and higher satisfaction with life. In addition, as the United Kingdom was a former colonial power of Sierra Leone, the relocation would be less difficult bureaucratically than for refugees from many other countries, and potentially more welcoming. Moreover, London, where all the participants were living, is a very cosmopolitan city, such that many nationalities integrate relatively easily. Also, due to the British education system having been imposed on Sierra Leone, many aspects of British life were already familiar to participants prior to their arrival. The combination of these factors contributes to an easier assimilation into the United Kingdom, and therefore the liminality of asylum seekers, as described in Sermpezis and Winter (2010), may have been avoided. As Thomas states:

> *The way of life in the UK is not completely different from Sierra Leone in the sense that Sierra Leone has been colonized by Britain. We have places in Sierra Leone like Liverpool Street. . . . I was in primary school and reading Charles Dickens . . . so I had that knowledge of Britain.*

In contrast to data from the narratives, safety did not appear as a superordinate construct in our repertory grid analyses, as demonstrated by analysis of the construct percentage sum of squares. This is surprising given the emphasis placed upon it in the Experience Cycle. Possible explanations for this are that safety had increased saliency when being discussed vocally and because the participants were to some extent reliving their experiences during discussion. Now that the participants are established in the United Kingdom and their safety is assured (and possibly taken for granted), safety has less urgency. That is, at a lower level of awareness (repertory grid analyses), participants placed less importance on safety compared to when they were consciously discussing it (Experience Cycle Methodology). Alternatively, repertory grid measurement of construct superordinacy may not be accurate, as currently debated in the literature (e.g., Fransella, Bell & Bannister, 2004). Safety was associated with the positive poles of constructs by all participants (see Chapter 2 regarding the bipolar nature of personal constructs). These were principally regarding happiness and strength. In addition, Farah, Mouna, and Simon also associated safety with good morals, kindness, and forgiveness.

It may be useful to note that all except Karimah and Thomas were, according to our analyses, of a low level of cognitive complexity. As higher cognitive complexity enables more accurate predictions (Bieri, 1955), this may have a bearing on results.

### Forgiveness and resilience

Leitner and Pfenninger (1994) argue that forgiveness is essential for optimal functioning. This could be extrapolated to being necessary for reconciliation, particularly in intra-national conflicts, where victims and perpetrators will live alongside each other after a war has ended. Forgiveness requires work by both parties, including acknowledging responsibility and committing to reconstruing in such a way as to avoid hurt reoccurring. Its importance to our participants was evident in narratives, as it emerged as an overarching theme.

> *You have to let go and forgive, otherwise you'll go mad just thinking about revenge . . . [it helps the] healing process.*

> (Thomas)

A degree of inconsistency was observed for several participants in expressing a will to forgive, particularly for the sake of peace, in the narrative but not in the repertory grid. This could be indicative of the repertory grid's ability to 'reveal aspects of construing at low levels of cognitive awareness, thus providing access to information which is unlikely to be revealed in an interview' (Winter, 1992, p. 65). It could also be demonstrating the ability of the repertory grid to identify where socially desirable responses have been supplied. Indeed the participants, being members of an NGO promoting community-based forgiveness, may actively be *trying* to forgive. All participants showed a degree of variation in their forgiveness, with unsurprisingly the lowest level observed during the war. Only in 10 years time did they think they would reach their original pre-war and ideal level of forgiving. This suggests there may be some form of temporal relationship, or lag time, between the committing of an atrocity and its forgiveness. As is well documented (e.g., Gillies & Neimeyer, 2006), coping with loss and bereavement is a complex and time-involving process. It may be this processing which is reflected in the temporal relationship. Indeed, Lopez-Lopez, Marin, Leon, Garzon and Mullet (2012) found that the willingness to forgive in Colombia, where a conflict was still ongoing, was much lower than that found in Lebanon, whose conflict had concluded over 20 years previously.

Consistent with their narrative data, Farah and Simon construed themselves as forgiving, with only minimal changes during the war and on arrival in the United Kingdom. In contrast, they construed war perpetrators as being unforgiving at all time points, with only very minimal improvement in 10 years time. This suggests they have difficulty in reconstruing war perpetrators, despite the passage of time and a conscious desire to forgive. Thomas showed the greatest variation in the construal of forgiveness over time, perhaps reflecting his higher cognitive complexity. In common with all participants, he was least forgiving during the war. However, unlike the others, he did not construe himself before the war as being as forgiving as his ideal self. This was further detailed in the narrative, where Thomas describes himself as becoming 'a better person' on joining a church in London. It is possible that he construes his current, Christian belief-based self as more forgiving than previously. Thomas also demonstrates more variation in his construing of war perpetrators. Karimah provided some intriguing and conflicting material. Despite her higher cognitive complexity, she displayed little variation in her construing of forgiveness: she construes war perpetrators as not forgiving at all time points but herself as forgiving before the war, now, and in 10 years. This is contradicted in the narrative, where she states that she is unable to forgive. Surprisingly, and worthy of further investigation, what may be thought of as the socially desirable response is present at a lower level of awareness, with the converse available more consciously. Forgiveness may hold great significance, or great difficulty, for Karimah. These findings are consistent with those of the amputee footballers in Chapter 6 and with recent research from Sierra Leone indicating that despite a personal and political desire for forgiveness, it is not always possible at a fundamental level (Brown, 2013).

Despite the dearth of research on the subject, forgiveness is of great value and concern. Not only is it important for optimal functioning, it can relieve psychological distress (Worthington, 1998), and it is also a 'principal contributing factor to resilience not only of individuals but also of societies recovering from major trauma' (Goins et al., 2012 , p. 21). In the repertory grid analyses of this study, however, the constructs of forgiveness and resilience were not closely correlated except for two participants, Farah and Thomas. This may be due to the complex difficulties associated with forgiveness, as described above, rather than a contradiction of Goins et al. (2012). Resilience mediates how individuals cope in the face of adversity, including conflict and migration. Studies have reported that resilience in the post-migratory environment has a stronger relationship with psychological morbidity than exposure to pre-migratory traumatic events (Gorst-Unsworth & Goldenberg, 1998).

Karimah, Mouna, and Shazia demonstrate a similar pattern of construing resilience: perceiving themselves as ideally resilient at all time points except during the war. They construed war perpetrators as the converse; being most resilient during the war and not at all after the conflict. It would appear that these participants have observed war perpetrators and their adaptation post-conflict, and have reconstrued them in terms of resilience, noting that this has decreased with the change in role from combatant to civilian. Thomas is of interest in that not only does he show most variation in construing, he does not construe himself at the ideal level of resilience at any time point. Once again, this could be a reflection of his higher cognitive complexity. However, it is also contradictory to his narrative, which supports the common theme of individual determination and stoicism. It is possible that whilst Thomas has a desire to be (and possibly a perception of being) resilient, this is not reflected at the fundamental level of his construct system.

> *It's an African thing . . . we just have to get on with life.*
>
> (Thomas)

Analysis of the narrative indicated that the role of religious belief was particularly important in resilience for all six participants.

> *But with God everything is possible . . . I knew that He would look after me.*
>
> (Mouna)

Religious beliefs are thought to provide psychological protection against adverse consequences (e.g., Holtz, 1998; Krotofil, 2013). In Australia, Islam provides an enduring 'home' for Somali refugees (McMichael, 2002). Religious awareness is therefore an important consideration in the resettlement of refugees (Whittaker et al., 2005) and is worthy of additional investigation.

Caution must be employed in generalizing the findings of this study. In addition to the small sample size, of primary importance is that the study investigated the movement of refugees to a developed country. In reality, less than a third of refugees do this (Carswell, Blackburn & Barker, 2011). The majority flee to neighbouring, underdeveloped countries where the prevailing issues and resources are likely to be somewhat different.

## Conclusions

Our study has revealed the multidimensional nature of forced migration and the intricacies of adjusting the personal construct system to life in a new country. This differs from the current main body of refugee literature that focuses on trauma-related psychopathologies. Findings here indicate that safety is of preeminent importance, appearing to be superordinate to all other constructions during forced migration. Individuals' construing of war perpetrators varies over time, with the exception of forgiveness, which appears fairly static. With narratives indicating a conflicting desire to forgive, the static value obtained from the repertory grid analysis suggests the opposite. It is proposed that civilians are unable to process forgiveness, despite a wish to do so, until a certain amount of time has elapsed, which could be interpreted as a 'forgiveness lag time'.

The practice of granting asylum to people fleeing persecution in foreign lands is one of the earliest hallmarks of civilization, with reference made to it in Assyrian texts written 3,500 years ago (United Nations High Commissioner for Refugees, 2013). Over three millennia later, the urgency of accommodating Syrian refugees remains prominent in the collective conscious. We need to reevaluate our roles as host societies, in order to facilitate the flourishing and resourcefulness of our refugee populations.

*I am not an Athenian or a Greek, but a citizen of the world.*

(Socrates, 469 BC–399 BC)

## References

Adhikari, P. (2012) The plight of the forgotten ones: Civil war and forced migration. *International Studies Quarterly,* 56: 590–606.

Bar-Tal, D. (2000) From intractable conflict through conflict resolution to reconciliation: Psychological analysis. *Political Psychology,* 21: 351–365.

Bellows, J., Miguel, E. (2006) War and institutions: New evidence from Sierra Leone. *The American Economic Review,* 96 (2): 394–399.

Berry, J. W. (1997) Immigration, acculturation and adaptation. *Applied Psychology: An International Review,* 46: 5–68.

Bieri, J. (1955) Cognitive complexity-simplicity and predictive behaviour. *Journal of Abnormal and Social Psychology,* 51(2): 263–268.

Braun, V., Clarke, V. (2006) Using thematic analysis in psychology. *Qualitative Research in Psychology,* 3(2): 77–101.

Brown, R. (2013) *'I fall down, I get up': Stories of survival and resistance following civil war in Sierra Leone.* Unpublished doctoral thesis, University of Hertfordshire, United Kingdom.

Burr, V., Giliberto, M., Butt, T. (2013) Construing the cultural other and the self: A personal construct analysis of English and Italian perceptions of national character. *International Journal of Intercultural Relations,* 39: 53–65.

Butt, T. (1996) PCP: Cognitive or social psychology. In J. W. Scheer, A. Catina (Eds.), *Empirical constructivism in Europe: The personal construct approach* (pp. 58–65). Giessen: Psychosozial-Verlag.

Butt, T. (2000) The person in society: Construct psychology and social action. In J. W. Scheer (Ed.), *The person in society: Challenges to constructivist theory* (pp. 176–185). Giessen: Psychosozial-Verlag.

Carlson, E. B., Rosser-Hogan, R. (1991) Trauma experiences, posttraumatic stress, dissociation and depression in Cambodian refugees. *American Journal of Psychiatry,* 148: 1548–1551.

Carswell, K., Blackburn, P., Barker, C. (2011) The relationship between trauma, post-migration problems and the psychological well-being of refugee and asylum seekers. *International Journal of Social Psychiatry,* 57(2): 107–119.

Davidson, G., Reser, J. (1996) Construing and constructs: Personal and cultural? In B. M. Walker, J. Costigan, L. L. Viney, B. Warren (Eds.), *Personal construct psychology: A psychology for the future* (pp. 105–128). Melbourne: Australian Psychological Society.

Epting, F., Prichard, S., Leitner, L. M., Dunnet, G. (1996) Personal constructions of the social. In D. Kalekin-Fishman, B. M. Walker (Eds.), *The construction of group realities: Culture, society and personal construct psychology* (pp. 309–322). Malabar, FL: Krieger.

Fazel, M., Wheeler, J., Danesh, J. (2005) Prevalence of serious mental disorder in 7000 refugees resettled in Western countries: A systematic review. *Lancet,* 365: 1309–1314.

Florczyk, S. (2014) *Does construing relate to acculturation attitudes and psychological well-being in Polish immigrants in the UK?* Unpublished doctoral thesis, University of Hertfordshire, United Kingdom.

Foucault, M. (1980) *Power/knowledge: Selected interviews and other writings, 1972–1977.* New York: Pantheon.

Fransella, F., Bell, R., Bannister, D. (2004) *A manual for repertory grid technique.* Chichester: Wiley.

Gillies, J., Neimeyer, R. A. (2006) Loss, grief, and the search for significance: Toward a model of meaning reconstruction in bereavement. *Journal of Constructivist Psychology,* 19(1): 31–65.

Goins, S., Winter, D. A., Sundin, J., Patient, S., Aslan, E. (2012) Self-construing in former child soldiers. *Journal of Constructivist Psychology,* 25: 1–27.

Gorst-Unsworth, C., Goldenberg, E. (1998) Psychological sequelae of torture and organized violence suffered by refugees from Iraq: Trauma-related factors compared with social factors in exile. *British Journal of Psychiatry,* 172: 90–94.

Guterres, A. (2005) *Message by U.N. High Commissioner for Refugees. World Refugee Day, 15 June 2005.* Available at: http://www.unhcr.org/cgi-bin/texis/vtx/search?page=search&docid=42afe7512&query=courage%20guterres [Accessed August 27, 2013].

Hardison, H. G., Neimeyer, R. A. (2012) Assessment of personal constructs: Features and functions of constructivist techniques. In P. Caputi, L. L. Viney, B. M. Walker, N. Crittenden (Eds.), *Personal construct methodology* (pp. 3–51). Chichester: Wiley-Blackwell.

Hobfoll, S. E. (1998) *Stress, culture and community: The psychology and philosophy of stress.* New York: Plenum.

Hobfoll, S. E. (2001) The influence of culture, community and the nested-self in the stress process: Advancing conservation of resources theory. *Applied Psychology: An International Review,* 50: 337–421.

Hollifield, M. H., Warner, T. D., Lian, N., Krakow, B., Kesler, J., Stevenson, J., Westermeyer, J. (2002) Measuring trauma and health status in refugees: A critical review. *Journal of the American Medical Association,* 288(5): 611–621.

Holtz, T. H. (1998) Refugee trauma versus torture trauma: A retrospective controlled cohort study of Tibetan refugees. *Journal of Nervous Mental Disease,* 186: 24–34.

Human Rights Watch (1999) *Sierra Leone: Getting away with murder, mutilation and rape.* New York: Human Rights Watch.

International Organisation for Migration. (2015) *Where we're from.* Available at: https://www.iom.int/world-migration [Accessed 2 August 2015].

Keen, D. (2005) *The best of enemies: Conflict and collusion in Sierra Leone.* Oxford: James Currey Ltd.

Kelly, G. A. (1955) *The psychology of personal constructs.* New York: Norton. (Reprinted by Routledge, 1991)

Kelly, G. A. (1963) *A theory of personality: The psychology of personal constructs.* New York: Norton.

Kelly, G. A. (1969) Man's construction of his alternatives. In B. Maher (Ed.), *Clinical psychology and personality: The selected papers of George Kelly* (pp. 66–93). London: Wiley.

Kelly, G. A. (1970) A brief introduction to personal construct theory. In D. Bannister (Ed.), *Perspectives in personal construct theory* (pp. 1–30). London: Academic Press.

Krotofil, J. M. (2013) Religion, migration and the dialogical self: New application for the personal position repertoire method. *Journal of Constructivist Psychology,* 26(2): 90–103.

Lazarus, R. S., Folkman, S. (1984) *Stress, appraisal and coping.* New York: Springer.

Leitner, L. M., Begley, E. A., Faidley, A. J. (1996) Cultural construing and marginalised persons: Role relationships and ROLE relationships. In D. Kalekin-Fishman, B. M. Walker (Eds.), *The construction of group realities: Culture, society, and personal construct theory* (pp. 323–340). Malabar, FL: Krieger.

Leitner, L. M., Pfenninger, D .T. (1994) Sociality and optimal functioning. *Journal of Constructivist Psychology,* 7: 119–135.

Lopez-Lopez, W., Marin, C. P., Leon, M.C.M., Garzon, D.C.P., Mullet, E. (2012) Columbian lay people's willingness to forgive different actors of the armed conflict: Results from a pilot study. *Psicologica,* 33: 655–663.

McMichael, C. (2002) 'Everywhere is Allah's place': Islam and the everyday life of Somali women in Melbourne, Australia. *Journal of Refugee Studies,* 15: 171–188.

Melander, E., Oberg, M. (2007) The threat of violence and forced migration: Geographical scope trumps intensity of fighting. *Civil Wars,* 9(2): 156–173.

Moore, W. H., Shellman, S. M. (2006) Refugee or internally displaced person? To where should one flee? *Comparative Political Studies,* 39 (5): 723–745.

Murray-Prior, R. (1998) Modelling farmer behaviour: A personal construct theory interpretation of hierarchical decision models. *Agricultural Systems,* 57: 541–556.

Oades, L. G., Patterson, F. (2016) Experience cycle methodology: A qualitative method to understand the process of revising personal constructs. In D. A. Winter, N. Reed (Eds.), *Wiley handbook of personal construct psychology.* Chichester: Wiley-Blackwell.

Oades, L. G., Viney, L. L. (2000) Experience cycle methodology: A new method for personal construct psychologists? In J. W. Scheer (Ed.), *The person in society: Challenges to constructivist theory* (pp. 160–173). Giessen: Psychosozial-Verlag.

Oades, L. G., Viney, L. L. (2012) Experience cycle methodology: Method for understanding the construct revision pathway. In P. Caputi, L. L. Viney, B. M. Walker, N. Crittenden (Eds.), *Personal construct methodology* (pp. 129–146). Chichester: Wiley-Blackwell.

Oliver, D. C., Schlutsmeyer, M. W. (2006) Diversity and multiculturalism in psychotherapy: A personal construct perspective. In P. Caputi, H. Foster, L. L. Viney (Eds.), *Personal construct psychology: New ideas* (pp. 99–108). Chichester: Wiley.

Ouarasse, O. A., Vijver, F.J.R. (2005) The role of demographic variables and acculturation attitudes in predicting sociocultural and psychological adaptation in Moroccans in the Netherlands. *International Journal of Intercultural Relations,* 29(3): 251–272.

Procter, H. (2016) Personal construct psychology, society and culture. In D. A. Winter, N. Reed (Eds.), *Wiley handbook of personal construct psychology.* Chichester: Wiley.

Rutter, J. (2003) *Supporting refugee children in 21st century Britain: A compendium of essential information.* Stoke-on-Trent: Trentham Books.

Ryan, D., Dooley, B., Benson, C. (2008) Theoretical perspectives on post-migration adaptation and psychological well-being among refugees: Towards a resource-based model. *Journal of Refugee Studies,* 21(1): 1–18.

Scheer, J. W. (Ed.) (2000) *The person in society: Challenges to a constructivist theory.* Giessen: Psychosozial-Verlag.

Scheer, J. W. (2003) Cross-cultural construing. In F. Fransella (Ed.), *International handbook of personal construct psychology* (pp. 153–161). Chichester: Wiley.

Sermpezis, C., Winter, D. (2010) The state of being in betwixt and between: Exploring the socio-temporal dimensions of asylum seeker and refugee trauma. In D. Bourne, M. Fromm (Eds.), *Construing PCP: New contexts and perspectives* (pp. 136–154). Norderstedt, Germany: Books on Demand.

Sewell, K. (2005) The experience cycle and the sexual response cycle: Conceptualization and application to sexual dysfunctions. *Journal of Constructivist Psychology,* 18: 3–13.

Silove, D., Franz, M. D. (1997) The psychosocial effects of torture, mass human rights violations and refugee trauma. *Journal of Nervous and Mental Disease,* 187: 200–207.

Stevens, Y. (2012) *Statement by the Sierra Leone Permanent Representative to the United Nations in Geneva.* International Organization for Migration 101st Council Meeting. 27–30 November 2012.

United Nations (2015) Department for Economic & Social Affairs, Population Division. Available at: http://esa.un.org/MigGMGProfiles/indicators/files/SierraLeone.pdf [Accessed 2 August 2015].

United Nations High Commissioner for Refugees (1975–2011) *Statistical Yearbooks, 1975–2011.* Available at http://www.unhcr.org/cgi-bin/texis/vtx/search?page=search&query=statistical+year+book&x=0&y=0 [Accessed 27 August 2013].

United Nations High Commissioner for Refugees (2013) *Global report 2012.* Available at: http://www.unhcr.org/gr12/index.xml [Accessed 27 August 2013].

Ward, C., Kennedy, A. (1999) The measurement of sociocultural adaptation. *International Journal of Intercultural Relations,* 23: 659–677.

Whittaker, S., Hardy, G., Lewis, K., Buchan, L. (2005) An exploration of psychological well-being with young Somali refugee and asylum-seeker women. *Clinical Child Psychology and Psychiatry,* 10(2): 177–196.

Winter, D. A. (1992) *Personal construct psychology in clinical practice: Theory, research and applications.* London: Routledge.

Winter, D., Patient, S., Sundin, J. (2009) Constructions of alienation. In L. M. Leitner, J. C. Thomas (Eds.), *Personal constructivism: Theory and applications* (pp. 171–189). New York: Pace University Press.

Wood, E. J. (2008) The social processes of civil war: The wartime transformation of social networks. *Annual Review of Political Science,* 11: 539–561.

Worthington, E. L. (Ed.) (1998) *Dimensions of forgiveness.* Philadelphia: Templeton Foundation Press.

# Part 3

# Implications

# Chapter 10

# Post-traumatic stress, growth and resilience

> *... There is no person without family, no learning without culture, no madness without social order; and therefore neither can there be an I without a We ...*
>
> (Martin-Baro, 1994, p. 41)

Chapter 2 highlighted and critically reviewed the theoretical and research literature on psychological responses to warfare and major trauma. What is clear from the developing literature and the stories shared in Part 2 is that people respond to the experience of trauma in multiple and complex ways, and it may not be helpful to attempt to find universal explanations to describe such experience. In fact, doing this may subjugate and oppress local ways of making sense out of experience and serve to perpetuate distress. This chapter will first consider further the three dominant Western conceptualizations of how people respond following trauma: post-traumatic stress, growth and resilience. The individual and collective constructing of trauma demonstrated through the stories in Part 2 will then be considered and learning highlighted. Specific critical reflection will then be given to the universal adequacy of Western concepts of such responses.

## 'Trauma and response'

The theoretical and research literature around individual and collective response following trauma indicates that a continuum of experience is evident, ranging from what may be considered 'normal' struggling, through to 'post-traumatic stress disorder', 'resilience or recovery', and 'post-traumatic growth'. Before discussing these constructs further it is useful to return to the definition of 'trauma' in Chapter 2 and broaden this discussion by considering the interconnected concept of 'response'.

'Trauma' is a term that is often employed in Western cultures to define and describe the distressing experiences that people encounter throughout life and their subsequent effects. The word 'trauma' is often used to describe both the event (e.g., war) and the effects or response (e.g., stress). The *Diagnostic and Statistical Manual (DSM-V)* (APA, 2013) describes trauma experiences as:

> exposure to actual or threatened death, serious injury or sexual violence in one or more of four ways: (a) directly experiencing the event; (b) witnessing, in person, the event occurring to others; (c) learning that such an event happened to a close family member or friend; and (d) experiencing repeated or extreme exposure to aversive details of such events, such as with first responders. Actual or threatened death must have occurred in a violent or accidental manner; and experiencing cannot include exposure through electronic media, television, movies or pictures, unless it is work-related.
>
> (p. 272)

Young (1995) locates the origins of the trauma discourse in the late nineteenth century, when the word 'trauma', previously understood as bodily damage, was extended to cover the psychogenic sequelae of distressing experiences. Weathers and Keane (2007) state that the usefulness of the idea as outlined in the *DSM*, that an event is only considered 'traumatic' if it is life-threatening, should be questioned. The experience of trauma around the world is diverse, and what may be considered traumatic to one person in one culture (for example, the loss of a house) may be considered a daily occurrence to another person in another culture. Some of the language now used in the literature includes 'continuous trauma', 'complex trauma' and 'compound trauma', and perhaps this is more reflective of contexts such as Sierra Leone.

Another important concept is that of the 'response' to adversity. This term is used to conceptualize how people cope and manage following adversity, how they respond. 'Response' is seen as a more useful construct than other concepts, for example 'effects', in order to honour the idea that, regardless of how people experience their lives after adversity, they will always *respond* in some way (Yuen, 2009). As White (2006) describes, people always take steps to endeavour to prevent or modify the trauma they are subject to or the effects it has on their lives. The concept of 'response' values the different ways people may manage and avoids potential judgements about what is a 'right' or 'wrong' reaction following adversity and trauma. This should be held in mind throughout the following discussion.

### Post-traumatic stress disorder (PTSD)

PTSD (Brewin, 2003) is currently the most publicly well-known distress response to adversity in Western society. Moghimi (2012) reviews how the PTSD label was first introduced into the Western psychiatric lexicon after the Vietnam War, which eventually led to the globalization of PTSD as the main cultural idiom for discussing trauma-related stress. As Chapter 2 describes, PTSD is discussed widely within the literature and research concerned with psychological responses following warfare and major trauma. As with many psychiatric constructs, there are both 'saviours' and 'sceptics' of the PTSD phenomenon (Brewin, 2003). A 'sceptical' argument is that PTSD is a product of the individualist and 'cognitive' culture in Western society. This perspective shows concern over the privileging of intrapsychic processes over and above the social context. From the 'saviour' position, a wide range of research, as discussed in Chapter 2, is offered which supports the claim that PTSD is an identifiable phenomenon. Some also suggest that the construct of PTSD is universal (Jobson & O'Kearney, 2009) and consistent across the few cultures that have been studied systematically (Brewin, 2003). However, Bracken, Giller and Summerfield (1995) highlight the fact that whilst symptoms and signs may be identified in different settings there is no guarantee that they mean the same thing. Furthermore, much of the research carried out in non-Western settings uses Western concepts (e.g., PTSD) as a frame of reference from which to study experience, for example, studies that aim to establish the occurrence of PTSD following warfare in a certain county; this is known as ethnocentric. Such a research design does not allow for alternative responses to be explored. Thus, research and understanding remains in a cycle that serves to privilege the Western constructs. As Goldsmith, Martin and Smith (2014) reflect, a narrow focus on PTSD may restrict funding for, and attention to, research that addresses other important antecedents and outcomes of trauma and thereby limit both scientific developments and potentially helpful interventions. The critical review presented thus far is not, as Bracken (1998) states, an attempt to deny the suffering that PTSD attempts to define. Rather, it proposes that the construct of PTSD is only one particular way of understanding such experiences. Bracken (1998) simply questions the ethics of using this construct to make sense of experiences *without* critical reflection.

## Post-traumatic growth

Aside from the developing criticism that PTSD is a socially constructed phenomenon, there is also analysis within the literature base which points out that PTSD is not the only way that people respond to trauma over time. Summerfield (2001) suggests that the discourse of 'the medicalized victim' in PTSD has become the most available story within Western society, meaning that other trajectories or responses may be more difficult to access. In support of this view, the Positive Psychology Movement (Joseph & Linley, 2008) within clinical psychology has criticized clinical psychology's focus on pathology. This view advocates that placing an emphasis on pathologizing people's experiences negates the opportunity to learn from individuals and groups who seem to be more resilient to life's challenges (Joseph & Linley, 2008).

Bracken (1998) highlights that the dominance of the PTSD model has cut off our view of other response trajectories. Recently the discipline of clinical psychology has been widening its focus to examine the different possible trajectories following adversity. Morland, Butler and Leskin (2008) identify positive trajectories such as when a person either maintains, returns to or exceeds their pre-trauma levels of functioning, whereas they view negative trajectories as presentations that involve disturbance, decline and permanent disability. 'The Feisty Survivor' is one positive trajectory which Summerfield (2001) believes has become subjugated in today's Western, 'illness-focused' society.

As Chapter 2 highlights, the phenomenon of post-traumatic growth (PTG) is a further construct which has been reported in the theoretical and research literature on psychological responses to warfare and major trauma. This construct has acquired numerous terms as the literature has developed, including growth following adversity, perceived benefits, positive aspects, transformation of trauma, construing benefits, stress-related growth, and flourishing (Tedeschi & Calhoun, 2004a). Terms have been used interchangeably, and there is not a single agreed collective term for this field of study (Linley & Joseph, 2004); however, it appears from the literature that post-traumatic growth is the most widely used. The idea that growth can follow suffering is an old concept, and evident in many world religions including Christianity, Buddhism, Hinduism, Islam and Judaism (Splevins, Cohen, Bowley & Joseph, 2010). Tedeschi, Park and Calhoun (1998) conceptualized growth following adversity as a significant beneficial change in cognitive and emotional life, which has behavioural implications. Further, they state that growth following adversity involves fundamental changes or insights about living and is not merely another coping mechanism. Linley and Joseph (2004) conceptualize growth as not simply the absence of post-traumatic stress, but rather an independent dimension of experience. Although the study of growth following adversity has largely developed separately from the study of PTSD, a number of researchers have highlighted that these two concepts are interconnected and can be understood within an integrative psychosocial framework (Joseph & Linley, 2008; Shakespeare-Finch & Lurie-Beck, 2014; Tedeschi & Calhoun, 2004a).

As Chapter 2 highlights, studies have reported growth following a range of adverse events, for example, bereavement, accidents and disasters, cancer, HIV and AIDS, sexual abuse, rape, illness, and war and conflict (Linley & Joseph, 2004). However, Splevins et al. (2010) highlight that, although studies have been carried out in a number of different countries, this multicultural evidence is based largely on quantitative data. It is also collected almost exclusively from one assessment tool: the Posttraumatic Growth Inventory (PTGI; Tedeschi & Calhoun, 1996). Splevins et al. (2010) make the argument that all the current measurement scales that aim to capture the phenomenon of post-traumatic growth are based on a Western, individualistic understanding. For example, items measuring changes in personal strength (e.g., changes in a feeling of self-reliance) incorporate an implicit assumption of the self as a distinct and separate entity. This may be strikingly different to belief systems held within collectivist cultures (Splevins et al., 2010). Three broad categories of growth are reflected in the currently available measurement tools: changes within relationships, view of self, and life philosophy (Joseph & Linley, 2006). However, Pals and McAdams (2004) highlight that people might experience growth in an area which does not fit into these predefined categories. One of the few qualitative studies completed within this area used participants of Australian nationality, and the results showed differences in the construction of growth from the commonly used PTGI. A more expansive compassion dimension and the absence of a spirituality/religiosity dimension was reported in this study (Shakespeare-Finch & Copping, 2007). Interestingly, Tedeschi and Calhoun (2004b) comment that they have not seen research which indicates that types of growth are reported other than those represented on the PTGI; however, lack of evidence cannot in itself provide evidence for validity. As Bracken et al. (1995) identify, while procedural norms based on Western epistemological and reductionist approaches towards science may be appropriate and meaningful for the populations within which they were developed, they may lead to culturally insensitive practices when applied to other cultures and communities. Such methodological issues highlight the need to consider how information is constructed. As Mishler (1991) demonstrates, survey questionnaires (such as the PTGI) can only measure what is being asked rather than take account of idiosyncratic narratives of the person being interviewed.

### Resilience

Alongside PTSD and PTG, the concept of resilience can be highlighted as the third dominant idea within theory and research around how people respond following warfare and major trauma. Resilience has been defined as the ability to maintain a relatively stable, healthy level of psychological functioning in the face of highly adverse events (Bonanno, 2004). Community resilience is defined as positive collective functioning after experiencing a mass stressor, such as a natural or human-made disaster. Building on this idea, Lepore and Revenson (2006) highlighted different aspects of resilience by delineating the ideas of recovery, resistance and reconfiguration. In this conception, *recovery* refers to a response when a person may be initially challenged by a stressor but is ultimately able to return to his or her original state following adversity. *Resistance* refers to a response when a stressor does not appreciably affect a person. Alternatively, their concept of *reconfiguration* refers to a response when a person makes a permanent adaptation or alteration as a consequence of adversity. In this framework it is the construct of *reconfiguration* that seems to be aligned most closely with what has been most commonly referred to as post-traumatic growth (PTG; Joseph & Linley, 2008). The difference between 'resilience' and 'growth' has been described as the idea that 'growth' represents a response that goes *beyond* a person's previous level of functioning (Joseph & Linley, 2008). However, as with PTSD and PTG, the idea of resilience following trauma cannot be understood as an individual intrapsychic process. Scholars increasingly assert that resilience must be understood within a framework that prioritizes the dynamic interaction between individuals and their social and political environments; seen this way, well-being depends on both individual and environmental factors (Betancourt & Khan, 2008; Shinn & Toohey, 2003; Ungar, 2013).

## Learning from Sierra Leone

A review of the theories underlying the constructs of PTSD, PTG and resilience was provided in Chapter 2. The overarching criticism is that to date the models underlying these concepts have failed to consider how a person's *political, historical, societal and cultural context* shapes their response. The dominant theories in academic literature focus on intrapsychic processes and fail to hold in mind the influence of individuals' interpersonal relationships and discourses held in their family and social context (Maercker & Horn, 2013).

Two clear underlying assumptions stand out within the theory and research around the constructs of PTSD, PTG and resilience: that the self is construed individually, and that trauma or adversity is unusual rather than a part of life. Part 2 of this book has outlined the results from a number of research studies that have been conducted in Sierra Leone over the last 10 years. Content from this research will now be considered in relation to the two highlighted assumptions that underlie the dominant constructs of how people respond following warfare and major trauma.

### Assumption: the 'self' as construed individually

There is a historical African philosophical principle meaning 'humanity to others', often explained within the phrase 'Ubuntu – I am because we are, and since we are, therefore I am' (Mbiti, 1969, p. 109). In his book *In Sierra Leone*, Jackson (2004) talks about how the Koranko tend to construct experience as intersubjective rather than intrapsychic and how, historically, in Africa, more emphasis has been placed on society rather than on the self. Not all cultures make sense of life from the standpoint of an individuated self. As Holdstock (2000) reflects, the sense of relatedness is indeed at the very root of individualism.

Chapter 8 discussed research findings that suggested that a key dilemma following the civil war was about whether life was managed by the community or on one's own: whether 'we bear it' (together) or 'I bear it' (alone).

One participant, Gladi, developed a significant storyline within her narrative regarding how her community came together to support each other.

RJB:    . . . what's life been like for people since the end of the war?
Gladi:   . . . Oh, the end of . . . Uhh, in . . . during the . . . the end of the war, in my community, I mean, we will . . . we all came together and formed a group so that we'll be helping each other. (Okay. Uhh huh) We created home share. We used to go to . . . it's (Pause) five, uhh, man committee. We used to visit . . . uhh, they used to visit me. (Pause) They will come to my place, (Pause) and pray with me, (Pause) having share . . . if I have food, we share together. Then the other day we go to other person. When anyone of us is sick, that's our concern. We pay a visit to the individual, yes. We have concern for each other.

At the end of the war, Gladi speaks about how people responded to the experience of civil war by coming together, sharing what they had, and helping each other.

Interestingly, another participant, Selina, shares a story about receiving help from Action Aid, where she refers to help being offered to '*the community, not I*', and she also makes reference to how '*everyone, not one, because everyone was a victim*'. Here again Selina developed a '*We bear it*' response storyline. However, she then almost contradicts this in her following phrase,

> *Everyone is on his own. (Everyone . . . ?) Doing things (Everyone) by herself or himself, or his family anyway. So I just have to say so . . . because everyone is doing good although things are hard. . . .*

(Selina)

It seems that within Selina's story, a tension was present between the dominant and cultural resource of '*I am because we are, therefore we bear it*', compared to perhaps the alternative counter narrative of '*I bear it*'. Interestingly, this counter narrative is still voiced through the framework of 'we' as indicated in the phrase '*everyone is on his own*' as opposed to '*I am on my own*'.

Within Abdou's narrative, he explained exactly how hard it is to forget the atrocities committed and, therefore, how people lost confidence in each other.

> *And before the war, everyone had confidence in each other, you see. You don't mind what people would say or what people would do, we just accept, you know. . . . People started losing confidence from each other. You are a rebel or you are really the rebel collaborator. You see. . . . Or you are a member of your family or even extended family they are rebel, [inaudible 00:04:26] these are because he's a rebel. You see, when there are atrocity people will go for you if you are making a nuisance. It's not working, you see. And by then the war was tense.*

(Abdou)

It comes across in Abdou's narrative that the reality of *survival* during and after the war was that people did not trust each other. Despite the values in society that may have been present before the war, the basic day-to-day need to survive meant that people had to learn to cope alone, and this has not been forgotten. This is similar to the story that Gabriel tells in his individual narrative. Gabriel shares a powerful story about how, after the war, people '*don't like each other*'; yet he also contradicts this within his narrative when he talks about how God has enabled communities to come together and live in peace. Through his story telling Gabriel demonstrates the difficulty of integrating his personal meaning-making (that everyone is on his own) with the more dominant cultural narrative (that it is *God* who has enabled everyone to be able to cope with life *together*).

*Yeah, before the war, we love ourselves. I can leave here and go to my friend's house. I can stay there for even one week, two weeks. . . . He will say, "Hey mister, there's a food here. Let's go and eat." Okay. We go together. We eat. Take money from the pocket. We share. There's nothing like differences. But now, Freetown is hard in the way . . . we don't even like ourselves anymore.*

(Gabriel)

In this storyline Gabriel speaks clearly of his view that society changed from a place where everyone shared what they had and loved each other into a hard place where no one likes the other; '*I bear it*'. Likewise, Chapter 6 depicts the healing power of belonging to a football team when you are an amputee and none of the rest of society acknowledge your existence.

*We join ourselves together to meet our interest . . . we feel happy, because we see ourselves together.*

(F4, aged 37, amputated aged 15)

As Hobfoll, Mancini, Hall, Canetti and Bonanno (2011) discuss, rather than the individuality observed in the Western world, people in traditional African societies focus their lives around the extended family and the kinship group. In the face of political violence, the availability of collective resources is often overwhelmed by the need for them among populations. Among populations suffering from political violence, recovery must happen not only within individuals but also within larger social and political contexts (Almedom & Summerfield, 2004). Yambasu (2002) discusses the African belief that every individual has a role to play in the universe, 'everything in relation', and people must strive to maintain a balance between a personal identity as a unique individual and a communal identity. It stands out that the stories told in the interviews described in Chapter 6 demonstrate individuals' attempts to negotiate a balance between the '*We*' and the '*I*'. This highlights that the assumption suggested to underlie the dominant models of PTSD, PTG and resilience, 'the "self" as construed individually', does not hold true from the data collected in Sierra Leone. Responding to trauma is not simply an intrapsychic process but one that has to be negotiated through interpersonal and societal relationships and within a social, cultural, political and historical context. Indeed, in Sierra Leone and beyond, perhaps responding to trauma and adversity is not so unusual.

### Assumption: trauma and adversity as unusual

*You call it a disorder my friend, we call it life.*

(Forna, 2010, p. 319)

In Sierra Leonean culture, pain is seen as an unavoidable part of life, and a person is expected to bear it (Jackson, 2004). Trauma and adversity are part of life rather than the unusual 'shattering' experience which is the assumption behind the dominant Western conceptualizations. The focus in Sierra Leone, for the majority, has always been survival and the meeting of practical needs. As this is being written, the virus Ebola is storming the country, and the need for survival is escalated beyond the day-to-day 'managing'. The focus on 'practical first' and simply getting on with life has a social and historical context in Sierra Leone. As Selina states within the research described in Chapter 8, 'You just sit down'. Unlike in the West, it is suggested that in Sierra Leone people may not have constructs which relate to a preexisting expectation that adversity is unusual or life-threatening events 'happen to other people'. They expect to have to 'bear life'. As has been discussed within the research described in Part 2, in Sierra Leone religion is a central construct that helps people to make sense out of life. In Sierra Leone, God is considered the ultimate cause of a person's fortune or misfortune in life and death, with the ultimate responsibility for everything.

> *Things change but seldom because of anything we do.*
>
> (quoted to Jackson, 2004, p. 9)

Chapter 9 presented the stories of six refugees who fled to England to escape the civil war. The results of this research indicated that safety was elicited as a construct in each participant's repertory grid. As Chapter 9 considers, despite the researcher's attempts to elicit additional constructs, each participant held a tight prediction that the United Kingdom would provide a safe refuge. This was in comparison to life in Sierra Leone as uncertain and violent.

> *They want to kill me . . . that's why I run away . . . and we are walking with no food for 20 days, no washing . . . you are walking for your life.*
>
> (Karimah)

As described in Part 1, Sierra Leone has experienced a long and violent history. The way survivors made sense out of experience is couched in this historical, political, societal and cultural context. As Thomas (research participant, Chapter 9) succinctly describes, 'It's an African thing . . . we just have to get on with life'.

Moghimi (2012) extends these ideas by highlighting that the focus of PTSD symptoms tends to be on past events; however, in a continuously deprived environment, an individual may be more preoccupied with the trauma of daily living. Moghimi goes on to state that continued living and exposure to trauma in post-conflict societies is a much different experience than that of Vietnam veterans who eventually made it back to safety. The dominant models that attempt to explain how people respond to trauma are based on unspoken narratives that trauma and adversity are not part of everyday living. The stories from Sierra Leone clearly contradict this assumption and therefore question the adequacy of these Western constructs.

> From a critical psychology perspective, all psychological work requires constant examination for what it reveals of relations of power and dominance.
>
> (Emerson & Frosh, 2004, p. 3)

## Conclusions

The discussion within this chapter has sought to provide an overview of the dominant conceptualizations about how individuals and collectives respond following trauma. The underlying assumptions of these constructs have then been considered in relation to the findings from research carried out in Sierra Leone and described in Part 2.

The aim of this critical discussion is not to suggest that the concepts of PTSD, PTG and resilience should be disregarded but rather to highlight that such descriptors need to integrate within their theory and models the relevance of cultural, historical, political and social context.

The cognitive orientation towards 'the self' and its assumptions about the meaning of reality are Western constructs (Bracken, 1998). Therefore, as Brewin (2003) tentatively suggests, the concept of PTSD may be useful in Western situations but perhaps not elsewhere. Bracken (1998) critically evaluates the current theories of PTSD and cites how different philosophers (for example, Wittgenstein and Heidegger) have questioned the idea that meaning is something generated 'cognitively' within individual minds. Instead, it is suggested that meaning is actually located in a public and social realm of language. This shifts attention away from the contents of individual minds and back to the social context. As Brewin (2003) points out, trauma does not only affect a person's beliefs, it also affects the person's socially constructed identity. Identity is contrasted against individual beliefs in that identity involves locating a person within his or her social world, not simply within the person's own mind.

In response to the critical review of the existing dominant paradigms described, Maercker and Horn (2013) proposed three levels as relevant interpersonal processes which should be adequately researched. First, the individual level comprises social affective states, such as shame, guilt, anger and feelings of revenge. Second, at the close relationship level, are social support, negative exchange (ostracism and blaming the victim), disclosure and empathy. Third, the distant social level represents culture and society, in which the collectivistic nature of trauma, perceived injustice and social acknowledgement are concepts that predict the response trajectories to traumatic stress. Furthermore, criticism of the development of the PTSD construct does not mean that sufferings from traumatic experiences are not real, but merely that something can be real and socially constructed at the same time (Moghimi, 2012).

Are Western conceptualizations adequate? No, not if they are used rigidly and positioned as 'truth' without due reflection on the context. Indeed, aside from lacking adequacy, there is a real risk that people whose intentions are benign may respond from an ethnocentric and imperialist position.

# References

Almedom, A. M., Summerfield, D. (2004) Mental well-being in settings of complex emergencies: An overview. *Journal of Biosocial Science,* 36: 381–388.

American Psychiatric Association (2013) *Diagnostic and statistical manual of mental disorders* (5th ed.). Arlington, VA: APA.

Betancourt, T. S., Khan, K. T. (2008) The mental health of children affected by armed conflict: Protective processes and pathways to resilience. *International Review of Psychiatry,* 20(3): 317–328.

Bonanno, G. A. (2004) Loss, trauma, and human resilience: Have we underestimated the human capacity to thrive after extremely adverse events? *American Psychologist,* 59: 20–28.

Bracken, P. (1998) Hidden agendas: Deconstructing post traumatic stress disorder. In P. Bracken, C. Petty (Eds.), *Rethinking the trauma of war* (pp. 38–59). London, New York: Save the Children and Free Association Books.

Bracken, P. J., Giller, J. E., Summerfield, D. (1995) Psychological responses to war and atrocity: The limitations of current concepts. *Social Science and Medicine,* 40(8): 1073–1082.

Brewin, C. (2003) *Post-traumatic stress disorder: Malady or myth?* New Haven: Yale University Press.

Emerson, P., Frosh, S. (2004) *Critical narrative analysis in psychology: A guide to practice.* Basingstoke, UK: Palgrave Macmillan.

Forna, A. (2010) *In the memory of love.* London: Bloomsbury Publishing.

Goldsmith, R. E., Martin, C. G., Smith, C. P. (2014) Systemic trauma. *Journal of Trauma & Dissociation,* 15(2): 117–132.

Hobfoll, S. E., Mancini, A. D., Hall, B. J., Canetti, D., Bonanno, G. A. (2011) The limits of resilience: Distress following chronic political violence among Palestinians. *Social Science & Medicine,* 72(8): 1400–1408.

Holdstock, T. L. (2000) *Re-examining psychology: Critical perspectives and African insights.* New York: Routledge.

Jackson, M. (2004) *In Sierra Leone.* Durham, NC, & London: Duke University Press Books.

Jobson, L., O'Kearney, R. T. (2009) Impact of cultural differences in self on cognitive appraisals in posttraumatic stress disorder. *Behavioural & Cognitive Psychotherapy,* 37(3): 249–266.

Joseph, S., Linley, A. (2006) Growth following adversity: Theoretical perspectives and implications for clinical practice. *Clinical Psychology Review,* 26(8): 1041–1053.

Joseph, S., Linley, A. (2008) *Trauma, recovery and growth: Positive psychological perspectives on posttraumatic stress.* Hoboken: Wiley.

Lepore, S., Revenson, T. (2006) Relationships between posttraumatic growth and resilience: Recovery, resistance, and reconfiguration. In L. G. Calhoun, R. G. Tedeschi (Eds.), *Handbook of posttraumatic growth* (pp. 24–46). Mahwah, NJ: Erlbaum.

Linley, A., Joseph, S. (2004) Positive change following trauma and adversity: A review. *Journal of Traumatic Stress,* 17: 11–21.

Maercker, A., Horn, A. B. (2013) A socio interpersonal perspective on PTSD: The case for environments and interpersonal processes. *Clinical Psychology & Psychotherapy,* 20(6): 465–481.

Martin-Baro, I. (1994) *Writings for a liberation psychology.* New York: Harvard University Press.

Mbiti, J. (1969) *African religions & philosophy.* Ibadan, Nigeria: Heinemann.

Mishler, E. G. (1991) *Research interviewing: Context and narrative.* New York: Harvard University Press.

Moghimi, Y. (2012) Anthropological discourses on the globalization of posttraumatic stress disorder (PTSD) in post-conflict societies. *Journal of Psychiatric Practice,* 18(1): 29–37.

Morland, A. L., Butler, L. D., Leskin, G. A. (2008) Resilience and thriving in a time of terrorism. In S. Joseph, A. Linley (Eds.), *Trauma, recovery and growth: Positive psychological perspectives on posttraumatic stress* (pp. 39–61). Hoboken: Wiley.

Pals, J. L., McAdams, D. P. (2004) The transformed self: A narrative understanding of post traumatic growth. *Psychological Inquiry,* 15(1): 65–69.

Shakespeare-Finch, J., Copping, A. (2007) A grounded theory approach to understanding cultural differences in posttraumatic growth. *Journal of Loss and Trauma,* 11(5): 355–371.

Shakespeare-Finch, J., Lurie-Beck, J. (2014) A meta-analytic clarification of the relationship between posttraumatic growth and symptoms of posttraumatic distress disorder. *Journal of Anxiety Disorders,* 28(2): 223–229.

Shinn, M., Toohey, S. M. (2003) Community contexts of human welfare. *Annual Review of Psychology,* 54: 427–459.

Splevins, K., Cohen, K., Bowley, J., Joseph, S. (2010) Theories of posttraumatic growth: Cross cultural perspectives. *Journal of Loss and Trauma,* 15(3): 259–277.

Summerfield, D. (2001) The intervention of post-traumatic stress disorder and the social usefulness of a psychiatric category. *British Medical Journal,* 322: 95–98.

Tedeschi, R. G., Calhoun, L. G. (1996) The post traumatic growth inventory: Measuring the positive legacy of trauma. *Journal of Traumatic Stress,* 9(3): 455–471.

Tedeschi, R. G., Calhoun, L. G. (2004a) Posttraumatic growth: Conceptual foundations and empirical evidence. *Psychological Inquiry,* 15(1): 1–18.

Tedeschi, R. G., Calhoun, L. G. (2004b) The foundations of posttraumatic growth: New considerations. *Psychological Inquiry,* 15(1): 93–102.

Tedeschi, R. G., Park, C. L., Calhoun, L. G. (1998) *Posttraumatic growth: Positive changes in the aftermath of crisis.* London: Routledge.

Ungar, M. (2013) Resilience, trauma, context, and culture. *Trauma, Violence, & Abuse,* 14(3): 255–266.

Weathers, F. W., Keane, T. M. (2007) The criterion a problem revisited: Controversies and challenges in defining and measuring psychological trauma. *Journal of Traumatic Stress,* 20: 107–121.

White, M. (2006) Working with people who are suffering the consequences of multiple trauma: A narrative perspective. In D. Denborough (Ed.), *Trauma: Narrative responses to traumatic experience* (pp. 25–85). Adelaide: Dulwich Centre Publications.

Yambasu, S. J. (2002) *Dialectics of evangelization: A critical examination of Methodist evangelization of the Mende people in Sierra Leone.* Accra, Ghana: AOG Literature Centre.

Young, A. (1995) *The harmony of illusions: Inventing post traumatic stress disorder.* Princeton, NJ: Princeton University Press.

Yuen, A. (2009) Less pain, more gain: Explorations of responses versus effects when working with the consequences of trauma. *Explorations: An E-Journal of Narrative Practice,* 1: 6–16.

# Chapter 11

# Mental health service provision

Much has been written about the dire need to scale up mental health services in general for low- and middle-income countries (LMIC) (Song, van den Brink & de Jong, 2013). However, the push for a parity between Western and non-Western countries comes in the context of critical concern about the globalization of dominant models of mental health and mental illness (Summerfield, 2004; Watters, 2010; White, 2013). The way that Sierra Leone as a country understands and seeks to manage individuals' and communities' experience of distress has occurred within the historical context of slavery, colonization, and civil war; where power belongs to the other. In comparison, Western countries' current understanding and ways of managing individuals' and communities' experience of distress have developed in a context of the scientific revolution, colonization (of the other), and general economic growth; power lies within.

This chapter will consider the ways Sierra Leone and other countries in postconflict situations currently support people experiencing distress. The debate and dilemmas about what would be best practice will be contemplated, with the concluding proposal that it is not useful to consider one approach as more 'right' than others; that the promotion of human rights is the bottom line; and that best practice must be locally driven. Before considering the existing provision in Sierra Leone and beyond, the different ideas (models) about why people experience distress will be briefly considered.

## What are the different ideas about why people experience distress?

Chapter 7 highlights the different explanatory models which service users, staff, and medical students use to explain the phenomenon of what we call mental health problems. Processes noted included 'too much thinking'; lack of practical resources, family and social support; drug and alcohol abuse; and evil spirits.

There are numerous different models, theories and ideas about why people experience distress and suffering during their lifetime. Some of these models and ideas draw from scientific paradigms, and some draw from spiritual and

existential frameworks; few manage to encompass both. The different explanatory frameworks have developed in historical, political and cultural contexts and
reflect, and have affected, the dominant discourses within particular societies at
certain points in time. It is a bidirectional process. A broad overview of three
explanatory models will now be considered in order to contextualize the following discussion. The three models described place an emphasis on trying to
understand the causation of distress, which is often referred to in Western societies as 'mental illness'. The focus of causation is placed within a different aspect
of the human experience (biological, psychological, social, spiritual). There is no
doubt that this overview could be criticized for privileging a Western lens; it is
a considerable challenge to leave one's own frame of reference entirely.

## Medical model

The medical model, based on causal determinism, holds that mental health
problems arise from biological origins (e.g., malfunctioning genes; neurotrans-
mitters). Like physical health problems, distress is seen as something that has
an identifiable biological cause, which if identified correctly can be treated
with medication to correct the malfunction. This explanatory framework
has led to the development of the diagnostic systems (DSM-V; ICD-10) that
dominate the statutory mental health systems in many Western countries.
However, numerous authors have questioned whether a medicine of the mind
can work with the same epistemology as a medicine of the tissues (Thomas,
Bracken & Yasmeen, 2007; Tyrer, 2012). These authors question how distress
can be understood without due attention being paid to local understandings,
values and beliefs.

## Psychosocial models

Psychological explanatory models of distress are multiple, but the overarching
framework holds that difficulties, or indeed experiences of well-being, are a
product of what happens to a person throughout his or her life. Interconnected
to psychological understanding of distress are social explanatory models. Social
models place the emphasis on the influence of societal (external) factors (e.g.,
poverty, inequality) on the life experiences of individuals and groups (Commission on the Social Determinants of Health, 2008; Marmot, 2013; Wilkinson &
Pickett, 2010). In comparison, psychological explanatory models tend to focus
on the internal working models of individuals (Bateman & Fonagy, 2012; Wells,
2013). However, the interconnectedness between internal working models and
societal discourses and environments is key. Psychosocial explanatory models see
the external social and internal psychological worlds of individuals and groups
as interacting. Through this framework, psychosocial models would hold that
changes in brain function, or indeed cognitive processes, may be a product of
unfair societies (Marmot, 2013) rather than the cause.

## Traditional/religious model

From a traditional/spiritual perspective, distress is seen as being connected to supernatural forces. To generalize, narratives tend to explain that there are good and bad forces in the world, and that suffering is a result of being possessed by the bad or through falling out of favour with the good through past behaviour. Furthermore, when God is seen as 'the ultimate controller', all experience is attributable to God's will. A study (Alghali, Nahim & Alghali-Kaitibi, 2013) of Sierra Leoneans' perceptions of mental health in 2002 found that 25 per cent thought psychological problems were due to substance abuse, 16 per cent cited 'God's will', and 10 per cent believed such conditions were associated with 'spirits, curses or demons'. Similar findings were highlighted in Chapter 7:

> It's common with Africans to solicit the help of juju men to hurt those they don't like, those they consider to be their enemy.
> (PH6M, male psychiatric hospital resident, aged 79 years)

When considered within an empirical framework, the traditional/religious model of understanding distress and providing treatment is criticized for not having an evidence base (mhLAP, 2012). Though there are few studies on traditional healers in Sierra Leone, one study described the important role they have in performing a body purification ritual for former child soldiers (Stark, 2006). Through this symbolic healing, the traditional healer can aid in the experience of being accepted by the community.

The importance of culture, society and ways of understanding will be explored in depth in Chapter 14. However, it is important to note now that explanatory models or ideas which attempt to explain and understand distress or mental illness are commonly based on the dominant beliefs in a certain society about what is 'normal' and what is 'abnormal', and what is acceptable and unacceptable behaviour. Models of distress are therefore socially constructed. In comparison, postmodernism advocates a diversity of views, known as epistemological pluralism, and multiple ways of knowing (Burr, 2003). Postmodernism, therefore, rejects the idea that there can be one truth, which is discoverable through scientific understanding.

This chapter will conclude by considering what would be best practice. Before returning to the dilemmas inherent within this question, the reality of the existing provision of mental health services in Sierra Leone and beyond will be examined.

# Mental health service provision in Sierra Leone

## Overall health structure

Sierra Leone is one of the world's poorest countries; ranked 177 out of 186 countries in the UN's Human Development Index. In 2014 the Central

Intelligence Agency (CIA) estimated average life expectancy in Sierra Leone was 57.39 years. Following the civil war between 1991 and 2002, the country's entire infrastructure was damaged, including its health systems. Medical care is generally charged for in Sierra Leone, and it is provided by a mixture of government, private, and non-governmental organizations (NGOs). The Ministry of Health and Sanitation is responsible for organizing health care. The Red Cross (2014) outlines the numerous diseases that Sierra Leoneans face stemming from health and sanitation issues: malnutrition, anaemia, neonatal infection, diarrhoeal diseases, pneumonia, and malaria are all common causes of infant deaths. The Red Cross (2014) also reports that only 40 per cent of the population has access to safe drinking water. Dirty water gives rise to waterborne diseases and ailments such as diarrhoea, hepatitis A, cholera and typhoid fever. Following the *Maternal Health Is a Human Right* campaign by Amnesty International, in April 2010, Sierra Leone launched 'Free Health Care Medical Insurance', a system of free health care for pregnant and breast-feeding women and children under five. The current Ebola crisis is now ravaging an unstable health structure and further exposing the under-resourced health system in West Africa. The Kings Sierra Leone Partnership (KSLP), which aims to help build Sierra Leone's health system by strengthening training, clinical services, policy and research, reports a critical shortage of nurses, dentists and allied health professionals and specialists, and fewer than 150 doctors working in the public sector (KSLP, 2014).

## Policy context

Until 2009 Sierra Leone had no mental health policy, except its outdated 'Lunacy Act of 1902'. The Sierra Leone Mental Health Policy (2009) was finally written by the government of Sierra Leone through the support of the World Health Organization. This is a nationally based document and covers a wider range of needs including increasing the human resource base, decentralization of mental health services and promoting community-based services to clients (mhLAP, 2012). The policy also has as part of its strategic plan the need to review the 1902 Lunacy Act, which takes no account of the human rights of service users. The Sierra Leone Mental Health Strategy (2014–2018), the implementation plan for the Sierra Leone Mental Health Policy (2009), was only released in January 2014.

## Current provision

As discussed in Chapter 7 and above, it is well documented (mhLAP, 2012) that the dominant beliefs in Sierra Leone and wider Africa fall within the explanatory model of traditional/spiritual understanding: the belief that 'mental illness' is caused by demons/evil spirits. WHO (2012) reports that stigmatization is a major issue in the area of mental health in Sierra Leone, and it affects every aspect of service delivery, including attendance at clinics, compliance with medication and particularly the availability of social support. One research effort in a Sierra Leone community found that the majority of inhabitants believed mentally ill people to be evil, violent, lazy, stupid, unable to marry or have children and unfit to vote (WHO, 2012). Mental illness in Sierra Leone is seen as either brought upon oneself as punishment for certain actions such as the breaking of taboos, or as being cast upon someone by spells and witchcraft. Consequently, the traditional, church and mosque leaders are seen as able to drive out such evil forces. Research has indicated that the majority of people would consult a traditional healer first if they or a family member were experiencing distress (mhLAP, 2012). As Bell (1991) remarks, arguing for a plurality of service provision including both traditional and Western approaches, there is a commonality of beliefs, values and symbols between traditional healers, clients and their relatives. It has been estimated that 80 per cent of health care needs in low-income countries are met by traditional practices (Song et al., 2013), and approximately 90 per cent of mental health patients in Sierra Leone are treated by traditional methods and through other forms of informal community care. There is no government-funded community care or integration of mental health services into developing primary care health provision, although community health officers obtain a limited amount of mental health training in a three-week course at Sierra Leone Psychiatric Hospital.

There is a clear divide within Sierra Leone between services provided from a traditional/religious model, informing the majority of the community-level informal mental health care in Sierra Leone, and services provided from a medical model. The situational analysis completed by mhLAP (2012) highlights the centralization of mental health care/services provided and how medical mental health institutions are seen as the 'last resort' and that the people of Sierra Leone struggle to access such services due to the attached stigma. A brief review of the main services that aim to work with people experiencing mental health difficulties in Sierra Leone is now outlined.

### The Sierra Leone Psychiatric Hospital (SLPH)

The Sierra Leone Psychiatric Hospital, formally called Kissy Lunatic Asylum, was opened by the British in 1847. The inscription above the entrance read,

> *Royal hospital and Asylum for Africans rescued from slavery by British valour and philanthropy*
>
> (Jackson, 2005, p. 23)

Bell (1991) points out that initially, colonial authorities needed a place to house persons disturbing the public, and the hospital received patients with 'psychiatric illnesses' from Sierra Leone and other British West African territories. According to Bell, as in Foucault's (1973) description of the functions of the asylum, it was an institution for social control. As the country became more urban, Kissy became a place for those suffering from such social maladies as drug addiction, alcoholism, social alienation and homelessness (Bell, 1991). Furthermore, Heaton (2008) notes how Vaughan's historical works on colonial mental asylums in Africa illustrate the extent to which such asylums became spaces for the definition of the 'African mind' as inferior to the European. Indeed, Jackson (2005) states that 'opening asylums was one of the European colonizers' earliest social reforms – like a glove on the iron hand.'

Most of the services offered at SLPH are based on the medical model. The Sierra Leone Mental Health Policy (2009) reported that, at this point in time, there was one retired consultant psychiatrist[1], one medical officer, two trained psychiatric nurses, limited substance abuse treatment and no capacity for community follow-up services or specialized therapy. The policy further states that, because supplies are not forthcoming (for example, at the time of writing there had not been a delivery of mattresses for some 13 years), care and hygiene are below expectation as compared to any general hospital. In 2013 it was reported that the Human Rights Commission of Sierra Leone (HRC-SL) noted grave concern about the status of patients and caregivers at SLPH. The issue of human rights is explored further below. The hospital has a capacity for 150 patients but currently accommodates less than 100 in seven male and two female wards, staffed by 55 nurses and untrained mental attendants. The Sierra Leone press regularly carries headlines such as 'Has everyone gone crazy at Kissy "Crace" Yard?' – in this case, after the murder of a girl and maiming of a boy by their father, who had absconded from the hospital – going on to ask, 'Has it not been said that one sometimes has to act crazily in order to cure a mad person?' (Mamboreh, 2011).

Despite reading a journalist's account that the hospital was 'like a scene from Dante's Inferno', one of us (David) was still unprepared for what he encountered when he first visited it five years after the formal declaration of the end of the civil war. During the war, it had been looted by the rebels, who had destroyed some of its buildings. While the government had provided some funding for rebuilding, generators and equipment, most of the new buildings (including one labelled a therapy centre) were empty and locked, and in the absence of fuel to run the generators, there was no electricity. This rendered useless the new computers that the government had provided for senior staff, and which therefore still remained in their packaging. Food and water were in short supply, and 75 per cent of the patients were kept in chains. Virtually the only treatment was the administration of very high doses of major tranquillizers, generally well past their 'use by' date, when patients were first admitted or became disturbed. As described by the hospital's psychiatrist, the doses concerned were so high that they 'would kill a Westerner'. Staff, the majority of whom were untrained, earned 155,000 leones[2] per month, and their attendance for work was very variable. This particularly applied to night staff, who, viewing their work as too dangerous in the absence of electric lighting, would often only go into their assigned ward to record their attendance in the ward book before going home and leaving the patients to their own devices (which sometimes included breaking their beds and using these as weapons against each other). In the view of one senior staff member, some of the staff 'behave like patients – screaming at each other and fighting'. This individual considered that such problems had increased as a result of envy, and because 'the African mindset is vindictive', when a few staff had been selected to go on a delegation to a mental health service in London. He said that 'there are two key words missing in this hospital – love and respect'.

The situation in which patients found themselves is vividly described in a letter that was handed to David when he visited one of the wards:

*Dear Sir,*

*I write on behalf of my fellow patients here at the hospital. . . . Sir we are tired of the chain method. It doesn't seem to be working. It just imposes more anger into us. This makes us go back to our old ways. We are human being so we must be treated with dignity. The feeding is poor we are served as if we are prisoners. We are tied up with no water for drinking some of our inmates even drink their urine . . . MAY GOD BLESS US ALL!!*

Faced with this situation, delegations from Barnet, Enfield and Haringey Mental Health Trust in the English National Health Service (including David in five delegations and Rachel in one of these) attempted over the years to provide some training for the hospital staff after a process of twinning between this Trust and the hospital. That the initial rather didactic approach that was used hardly appeared to lead to fundamental changes in practice was indicated by comments on staff feedback forms such as that after the training they had lengthened patients' chains! A more consultative approach was therefore taken, involving discussion of challenging cases. However, the difficulties encountered in this are illustrated in the following interaction concerning a teenage boy (Winter, 2016, p. 195):

| David: | *Why is he in chains?* |
| Staff Member: | *He is usually fine but when we give him the medication he becomes disturbed, and then we have to put him in chains.* |
| David: | *So why do you give him the medication?* |

The staff member's response to this question indicated that he thought that David had taken leave of his senses! Nevertheless, he was persuaded to discuss the history of the boy's depression, which appeared to date from the disappearance, and probable death, of his father during the war. Staff were encouraged to talk to the boy about this history as an alternative to his current treatment regime of major tranquillizers followed by shackling.

The change in approach of the delegation also included each member of the delegation 'adopting' a ward. In David's case, this was a male ward with the highest number of chained patients in the hospital, and initially he was at a loss as to how to effect any change. He then remembered George Kelly's (1955) 'first principle' that 'if you do not know what is wrong with a person, ask him; he may tell you' (pp. 322–323). He therefore asked each patient on the ward not only what was wrong with him but also what might make his situation better if some change could be introduced on the ward. Apart from a former combatant who asked for war films to be screened, the patients almost invariably requested music. The delegation therefore bought a cassette player, staff agreed to bring in some of their cassettes, and when the music was first turned on, the patients spontaneously began to dance, albeit constrained by their chains. The staff were persuaded to unlock the chains of most of the patients, who then danced, holding their chains, with the staff. It was hoped that this intervention, together with those instituted on other wards by members of the delegation, would facilitate staff awareness of the humanity of their patients and would reduce the distance between them while minimizing the threat which, as we have seen in Chapter 7, this might pose.

During the course of the delegation's six visits to the psychiatric hospital over as many years, the number of in-patients kept in chains reduced to about 20 per cent. Although it is possible that the delegation's work contributed to this, the difficulty of sustaining change in a situation of annual visits was all too apparent. On one of the early visits, it came to the delegation's attention that the first lady of Sierra Leone (the newly elected president's wife) was a psychiatric nurse who had trained at the Institute of Psychiatry in London, but had never practised in her home country. We therefore asked if she could be invited to visit the hospital and open the therapy centre that had never been used but for which the delegation bought equipment. This request was greeted with scepticism since it was considered that she would be far too busy, but to our surprise on the day that we were due to fly back to London, we received a telephone call to say that she would attend, although only for 20 minutes. The staff duly lined the path along which she and her entourage walked to the therapy centre, where she opened it by cutting a ribbon and then gave an impassioned speech. She remained for some two hours, during which she chatted with some of the patients. The therapy centre is now named after her, with a new plaque announcing that it is the 'Sianyamah Koroma Therapy Department', but on our next visit we discovered that it was once again locked, and that its windows had been broken, with some of the equipment that we had bought having been stolen. By contrast, another building that was very much still in use was one labelled 'Cell', in which troublesome patients were chained in grim isolation.

We shall return in Chapters 14 and 15 to the appropriateness or otherwise of attempting to implement sustainable change by a system of occasional input by Western 'experts'.

## City of Rest (CoR)

CoR is a faith-based voluntary organization, which was established by a Christian pastor,[3] who had been working with drug addicts, in 1985 after he had a vision. As he said, 'God told me to do it.' In 2013, it moved from the centre of

Freetown to new premises on the outskirts on a site donated by the government, where, as well as sections for youths, women, and men, there is a large vegetable garden. It caters mainly to those identified as mentally ill and substance abusers, both Christian and Muslim. It is the only private residential service provided in the entire country (mhLAP, 2012), and although it can accommodate 70 residents, and has a current waiting list of 180, staffing levels in 2014 were only sufficient to cater for 42 'guests'. These are expected to pay 300,000 leones[4] a month, but those who are destitute (currently about 40 per cent) are exempted from this. Apart from this income, the institution relies upon donations. Its staff earn the equivalent of about £30 per month. Although, as in the psychiatric hospital, chaining is used and medication is administered, the regime also includes prayers, chanting, teaching, counselling, discussion groups and occupational therapy.

### Community Association for Psychosocial Services (CAPS)

CAPS (http://capssierraleone.weebly.com) offers individual and group psychosocial and physical rehabilitation services to community stakeholders and those who have suffered and survived trauma and torture. The organization also works to raise general awareness about trauma and psychosocial issues. It is the only local organization that provides psychosocial and physical interventions for torture and trauma survivors at all levels of the country. CAPS operates in the western and eastern provinces in Sierra Leone (that is, Freetown, Kono and Kailahun).

## Human rights

The shackling of people with mental health problems is particularly unfortunate in a country that was the home of freed slaves, although arguably it is not much less humane than some of the methods that have been used in the Western world with such individuals. That it is also likely to be counterproductive is indicated by Philippe Pinel's description of the unchaining of inmates of the Bicêtre and Salpêtrière asylums in Paris at the end of the eighteenth century. Thus, in regard to the effect of this on those who were unchained, he wrote that 'It is very important to note this improvement in the patients: it was a consequence of their liberation and better attitudes; if harsh treatment is used and enchainment continued dangerous hatred builds up leading to vengeful acts when least expected' (Pinel, 1995, p. 434). This is consistent with the account in the letter from a chained patient that was presented earlier in this chapter. Interestingly, Pinel also 'noted that some patients did not want their chains removed, it seems that they had got so used to having them on'. From a personal construct theory perspective, for these individuals (perhaps like many others in metaphorical chains throughout the world) being chained had become their 'way of life' (Fransella, 1970), and the unfamiliarity of, and new possibilities offered by, freedom were anxiety provoking. An editor's note to the original publication, in 1823, of Pinel's account states that 'it is hard to believe that there are still hospitals in several countries where this inhumane custom still exists'. He would hardly have countenanced that nearly 200 years later this practice would still be continuing.

The World Health Organization (WHO) endorsed mental health as a universal human right and a fundamental goal for health care systems of all countries (WHO, 2011). The Universal Declaration of Human Rights (United Nations, 2015) states,

> Everyone has the right to life, liberty and security of person; No one shall be held in slavery or servitude; slavery and the slave trade shall be prohibited in all their forms; No one shall be subjected to torture or to cruel, inhuman or degrading treatment or punishment.

Whilst some traditional healers may provide valuable support to individuals and communities experiencing distress, some of the traditional belief systems in Sierra Leone can be appraised as contributing to abusive treatment practices that fail to adhere to fundamental human rights. This is graphically depicted through Robin Hammond's photojournalism project '*Condemned*', which captures how people in Africa who experience mental distress are abandoned by governments, forgotten by the aid community, and neglected and abused by entire societies. Hammond graphically captures how Africans considered to be mentally ill are consigned to the dark corners of churches, chained to rusted hospital beds, or locked away to live behind the bars of filthy prisons (Hammond, 2013). Indeed, the practice of chaining within the Sierra Leone Psychiatric Hospital and the City of Rest (as described in the previous section), where more 'Western' styles of intervention are also administered, can also be questioned within the context of human rights. There are also movements, one example of which is the Citizens Commission on Human Rights (CCHR), which believe that the use of psychiatric medication, in both high-resource and low-resource countries, is nothing more than an invisible form of chaining and thus an abuse of human rights. The recently established National Mental Health Coalition is using the WHO Quality Rights toolkit to review the current situation in Sierra Leone's institutions and community services providing mental health care in order to bring about necessary reform.

## Is it just Sierra Leone?

The description of mental health provision in Sierra Leone is not dissimilar to that in many other African countries. Burns (2011) describes how services for mental illness and disability are inadequate across most of the continent. Most low-income/resource countries do not have mental health legislation or policies to direct relevant programmes, lack appropriately trained mental health personnel and are constrained by the prevailing public-health priority agenda and its effect on funding (Jack-Ide, Uys, & Middleton, 2012). As Burns (2011) highlights, where mortality is still mostly the result of infectious diseases and malnutrition, the morbidity and disablement due to mental illness receive very little attention from the government. Song et al. (2013) identified that the main barrier to care was a lack of government support, associated resource constraints and poor communication between and among government and local organizations.

Kigozi, Ssebunnya, Kizza, Cooper and Ndyanabangi (2010) report that Uganda's mental health legislation is outdated and offensive; the system operates on a mental health law that was last revised in 1964. The legislation focuses on custodial care of mentally ill persons and is not in accordance with contemporary international human rights standards regarding mental health care. Furthermore, the legislation was found to have a number of shortcomings such as failure to distinguish voluntary and involuntary care, inadequate protection and promotion of the human rights of people with mental illness, and the presence of derogatory and stigmatizing language (Kigozi et al., 2010). Services in Uganda remain significantly underfunded (with only 1 per cent of the health expenditure going to mental health) and skewed towards urban areas. Only 0.8 per cent of the medical doctors and 4 per cent of the nurses specialized in psychiatry (Kigozi et al., 2010). A further example is South Sudan. In 2014 the BBC reported how basic South Sudan's mental health system is; with only two psychiatrists and no mental health hospitals, people with mental health problems are kept in prison because there is nowhere else safe enough to house them. Whilst appraising the mental health systems in other African countries, it must be remembered that these reviews have been written by researchers from high-resource countries where medical models dominate. Therefore, the reviews are appraising African systems through the lens of what is considered best practice in high-resource countries, rather than perhaps a more culturally considerate analysis of such contexts.

## Recent developments

Whilst the health and mental health situation in Sierra Leone is extremely challenging and deeply concerning, there are two recent developments which are starting to shift the landscape: the Enabling Access to Mental Health Programme, and the Mental Health Coalition. The Enabling Access to Mental Health Programme aims to improve the quality of life and treatment available for people with mental health challenges in Sierra Leone through capacity building, advocacy and community sensitization. In 2011, the Mental Health Coalition of Sierra Leone was established, bringing together a wide range of government organizations, NGOs, religious groups, campaigners, mental health service providers, medical specialists and traditional healers. Jointly, these groups aim to raise awareness, push for a greater national commitment to mental health issues, and are currently petitioning the government to review the Lunacy Act of 1902 and offer greater protections for people with 'mental illnesses'.

These two movements have led to improved coordination and communication between the multiple organizations that aim to address the mental health needs within Sierra Leone. An observable outcome has been the development of a diploma course in psychiatric nursing through the College of Medicine and Allied Health Sciences, although the first graduates of this course have reported obstacles to being able to practise in their new roles. Furthermore, the Mental Health Coalition is pursuing ways in which financial support could be mustered to help train the two medical doctors who had opted for psychiatry training. A further current initiative is CONNECT Sierra Leone, a NGO based in Freetown that aims to support Sierra Leoneans working in the field of mental health overseas to repatriate to Sierra Leone and contribute to the development of an integrated, sustainable mental health service in the country.

The dilemma that is faced is that we know that the current mental health provision in Sierra Leone and other African countries is inadequate, and we know that some aspects or the treatment interpretation of current belief systems led to an abuse of human rights, but is embedding the Western medical model of mental health best practice or indeed ethical?

## What would be best practice?

Numerous researchers and academics (Marmot, 2013; Wilkinson & Pickett, 2010) have highlighted the roots of mental health problems as centred within the social environment; for example, in the case of Sierra Leone, the population's experience of warfare and ongoing poverty. As discussed throughout this book, much interest has centred on why some people develop difficulties following warfare and major trauma and why some people seem 'resistant' or indeed 'thrive' through the experience of adversity. What is clear through this discussion is that the different ways individuals and communities respond cannot be solely or primarily accounted for by an individualized medical model. Consequently, is it ethical for the global mental health movement to position Western models of mental health provision, many of which are dominated by the medical model and diagnostic systems, as best practice in low- and middle-income countries?

It has been reported that there is a current crisis within psychiatry (Tyrer, 2012). A developing research base is showing that with the exception of organic brain syndromes, there is no convincing empirical evidence that psychiatric disorders have a biological basis, and that therefore the evidence base for psychiatric medication is questionable (Speed, Moncrieff and Rapley, 2015; Tyrer, 2012). Research is also demonstrating that what actually influences the degree of mental ill health within countries is the degree of inequality between the richest and the poorest (Wilkinson & Pickett, 2010). To build on this, the research presented in Chapter 8 describes how distress within the trajectories of response narratives following the civil war in Sierra Leone was linked to the interplay between the dominant discourses in society and individuals' construing of events. What the community says about how one should be and manage, and how this compares to individual construing, matters; and what matters even more is whether individuals have some vehicle to negotiate discrepancies. This suggests that rather than 'scaling up' mental health services to be in line with Western services, programmes should both tackle human rights abuse *and* build on locally accepted and available strategies, targeting locally derived priorities and 'enabling communities'. Local understandings of mental health difficulties are often positioned as ignorant, and health promotion is advocated (Alghali et al., 2013). Just because some interpretations of traditional beliefs can lead to human rights abuse, this does not mean that all local understandings hold no value. Who has the power to decide what is the most useful model concerning mental health?

## Who is ignorant?

White (2013) has provided a comprehensive review of the wide-ranging concerns regarding the globalization of mental illness. Further critical discussion about the global mental health movement in an African context and lessons learnt from the research completed in Sierra Leone will unfold through Chapters 14 and 15. As Summerfield (2001) stresses, we must guard against assumptions that indigenous concepts of mental health difficulties are based on ignorance. Indeed, studies indicate that the prognosis for 'major mental health problems' is much better in less 'developed' countries than in the Western world (Warner, 2004). Instead, we should embrace ways of working which privilege local resources and offer the opportunity for facilitation rather than domination. Patel (1998) makes a similar point: 'Instead of attempting to change the explanatory models of entire communities to come in line with those of a largely hospital based biomedical psychiatry, it would be more pragmatic to adapt the psychiatric approach to [common mental disorders] to fit the models and beliefs already existing in the community' (p. 103). The Connecting People project funded by the National Institute for Health Research (NIHR) School for Social Care Research is a good example of such practice. Furthermore, White (2013) highlights how different disciplines need to come together and engage in constructive dialogue. This conversation should aim to develop cross-cultural understanding about how to meet the 'mental health' needs of people across the globe. As Jackson (2004) emphasizes,

> the situation of the other may be seen, not simply as one we want to save them from, making them more like us, but one we might learn from, even if this means greater acceptance of the suffering in this world, less crusading talk about how we may set the world to rights, and a place for silence.
>
> (p. 57)

## Conclusion

This chapter has considered the current mental health service provision in Sierra Leone and other African countries. Attention has been paid to the political context of such provision and the fundamental issue of human rights in relation to different belief structures. The question of 'what would be best practice?' has been grappled with and the idea of collaboration rather than domination has been reinforced as an overarching principle that should be core to any attempts made to 'improve' mental health provision in countries such as Sierra Leone.

## Notes

1  Dr. Edward Nahim, who also runs an outpatient clinic in Freetown.
2  About £24.
3  Pastor Ngobeh.
4  About £47.

## References

Alghali, S.T.O., Nahim, E. A., Alghali-Kaitibi, A. F. (2013) Health promotion as part of a holistic approach to community mental health care in Sierra Leone. *Sierra Leone Journal of Biomedical Research,* 5(1): 34–43.

Amnesty International (2010) *Maternal health is a human right.* Available at: http://www. amnestyusa.org/our-work/campaigns/demand-dignity/maternal-health-is-a-human-right [Accessed 12 March 2015].

Bateman, A. W., Fonagy, P. (Eds.) (2012) *Handbook of mentalizing in mental health practice.* Arlington, VA: American Psychiatric Association.

BBC (2014) *A South Sudanese psychiatrist's Herculean task.* Available at: http://www.bbc. co.uk/news/world-africa-29823344 [Accessed 3 February 2015].

Bell, L. V. (1991) *Mental and social disorder in sub-Saharan Africa: The case of Sierra Leone, 1787–1990.* New York: Greenwood Press.

Burns, J. K. (2011) The mental health gap in South Africa: A human rights issue. *Equal Rights Review,* 6: 99–113.

Burr, V. (2003) *Social constructionism.* London: Routledge.

CIA (2014) *The world factbook.* Available at https://www.cia.gov/library/publications/the-world-factbook/rankorder/2102rank.html [Accessed 25 June 2014].

Commission on the Social Determinants of Health (CSDH) (2008) *Closing the gap in a generation: Health equity through action on the social determinants of health.* Geneva: World Health Organization.

Foucault, M. (1973) *Madness and civilization: A history of insanity in the age of reason.* New York: Vintage.

Fransella, F. (1970) Stuttering: Not a symptom but a way of life. *International Journal of Language and Communication Disorders,* 5: 22–29.

Hammond, R. (2013) *Condemned – Mental health in African countries in crisis.* Available at: http://www.robinhammond.co.uk/condemned-mental-health-in-african-countries-in-crisis/ [Accessed 22 November 2014].

Heaton, M. M. (2008) *Stark roving mad: The repatriation of Nigerian mental patients and the global construction of mental illness, 1906–1960.* United States: ProQuest.

Jack-Ide, I. O., Uys, L. R., Middleton, L. E. (2012) A comparative study of mental health services in two African countries: South Africa and Nigeria. *International Journal of Nursing and Midwifery,* 4(4): 50–57.

Jackson, L. (2005) *Surfacing up: Psychiatry and social order in colonial Zimbabwe, 1908–1968.* New York: Cornell University Press.

Jackson, M. (2004) *In Sierra Leone.* Durham, NC, & London: Duke University Press Books.

Kelly, G. A. (1955) *The psychology of personal constructs.* New York: Norton. (Reprinted by Routledge, 1991)

Kigozi, F., Ssebunnya, J., Kizza, D., Cooper, S., & Ndyanabangi, S. (2010) An overview of Uganda's mental health care system: Results from an assessment using the world health organization's assessment instrument for mental health systems (WHO-AIMS). *International Journal of Mental Health Systems,* 4(1): 1.

KSLP (2014) *Health partnerships: Sierra Leone.* Available at: http://www.kcl.ac.uk/lsm/research/divisions/global-health/partnerships/sierraleone.aspx [Accessed 12 March 2015].

Mamboreh (2011, 24 March) Has everyone gone crazy at Kissy 'Crace' Yard? *New Storm,* p. 3.

Marmot, M. (2013) Fair society, healthy lives. In N. Eyal, S. A. Hurst, O.F. Norheim, D. Wikler (Eds.), *Inequalities in health: Concepts, measures, and ethics* (pp. 282–299). Oxford: Oxford University Press.

Mental Health Leadership and Advocacy Programme (mhLAP) (2012) The Sierra Leone Mental Health Policy cited in 'Report on Sierra Leone Situational Analysis'. Available at: https://enablingaccesstomentalhealthsl.files.wordpress.com/2013/04/situational-analysis-final-mhlap-sierra-leone-1-10-12_word.pdf [Accessed 12 March 2015].

Patel, V. (1998) *Culture and common mental disorders in sub-Saharan Africa.* Hove: Psychology Press.

Pinel, P. (1995) On the removal of chains from the insane. *Psychiatric Bulletin,* 19: 434 (originally published in 1823 in Archives Général de Médicine).

Red Cross (2014) *Health care in Sierra Leone.* Available at: http://www.redcross.org.uk/What-we-do/Health-and-social-care/Health-issues/Community-healthcare/Healthcare-in-Sierra-Leone [Accessed 12 March 2015].

Song, S. J., van den Brink, H., de Jong, J. (2013) Who cares for former child soldiers? Mental health systems of care in Sierra Leone. *Community Mental Health Journal,* 49(5): 615–624.

Speed, E., Moncrieff, J., Rapley, M. (Eds.) (2015) *De-medicalizing misery II: Society, politics and the mental health industry.* London: Palgrave Macmillan.

Stark, L. (2006) Cleansing the wounds of war: An examination of traditional healing, psychosocial health and reintegration in Sierra Leone. *Intervention,* 4(3): 206–218.

Summerfield, D. (2001) The intervention of post-traumatic stress disorder and the social usefulness of a psychiatric category. *British Medical Journal,* 322: 95–98.

Summerfield, D. (2004) 12 cross-cultural perspectives on the medicalization of human suffering. In G. Rosen (Ed.), *Posttraumatic stress disorder: Issues and controversies* (pp. 233–246). Chichester: Wiley.

The Sierra Leone Mental Health Strategy (2014–2018) Available at: http://www.mindbank.info/item/4287 [Accessed 12 March 2015].

Thomas, P., Bracken, P., Yasmeen, S. (2007) Explanatory models for mental illness: Limitations and dangers in a global context. *Pakistan Journal of Neurological Science,* 2: 176–177.

Tyrer, P. (2012) The end of the psychopharmacological revolution. *British Journal of Psychiatry,* 201(2): 168.

United Nations (2015) *The Universal Declaration of Human Rights.* Available at: http://www.un.org/en/documents/udhr/ [Accessed 3 February 2015].

Warner, R. (2004) *Recovery from schizophrenia: Psychiatry and the political economy.* Hove: Psychology Press.

Watters, E. (2010) *Crazy like us: The globalization of the American psyche.* New York: Simon and Schuster.

Wells, A. (2013) *Cognitive therapy of anxiety disorders: A practice manual and conceptual guide.* Chichester: Wiley.

White, R. (2013) The globalisation of mental illness. *The Psychologist,* 26(3): 183–185.

WHO (2011) *No health without mental health.* Available at: https://www.gov.uk/government/uploads/system/uploads/attachment_data/file/213761/dh_124058.pdf [Accessed 3 February 2015]

WHO (2012) *WHO proMIND: Profiles on Mental Health in Development.* Available at: http://www.who.int/mental_health/policy/country/sierra_leone_country_summary_2012.pdf [Accessed 12 March 2015].

Wilkinson, R., Pickett, K. (2010) *Spirit level* (2nd ed.). London: Allen Lane.

Winter, D. A. (2016) Transcending war-ravaged biographies. In D. A. Winter, N. Reed (Eds.), *Wiley handbook of personal construct psychology.* Chichester: Wiley-Blackwell.

# Chapter 12

# Perpetration of violence

The stories that have been told in this book have included accounts of almost unimaginable, and often seemingly gratuitous, violence, at times apparently designed to create the greatest possible suffering, both physical and psychological, in its victims. As has been noted in Chapter 6, acts such as those described are by no means specific to the civil war in Sierra Leone, or indeed to conflicts between people in the less 'developed' world, despite sometimes being portrayed as such. To view them as alien may serve the purpose of dissociating ourselves from the threatening possibility that we, under comparable circumstances, could act in a similar way, but it ultimately forecloses any prospect of understanding how one human being could subject others to atrocities of the sort that our participants have described. This chapter aims to facilitate such an understanding.

As we have seen, George Kelly's (1955) personal construct psychology stresses the importance in interpersonal relationships of 'sociality', attempting to see the world through the other's eyes. Kelly also advocated that personal construct psychologists should take a 'credulous attitude', taking the stance that 'From a phenomenological point of view the client – like the proverbial customer – is always right' (p. 322). This does not necessarily mean accepting the other person's view of his or her world, but it does mean taking that view seriously. Credulity may be stretched to its limits when applied to someone who has engaged in acts of extreme violence, but nevertheless there have been attempts to adopt a personal construct approach in attempting to understand such individuals (Horley, 2003; Houston, 1998; Winter, 2007). We shall provide brief examples of some of this previous work before considering how it may elucidate the experience of perpetrators of violence in conflicts such as that in Sierra Leone.

## Understanding perpetrators of extreme violence

### Serial killing

For Kelly, all behaviour is an experiment designed to test out the individual's constructions of the world. Killing, as a behaviour, is no exception, and if one killing is regarded as an experiment, serial killing can be seen as the killer's research programme. The book written by a British serial killer, Ian Brady, on his specialist subject of serial killing has provided an indication of how this programme is developed, allowing the individual to elaborate their 'career' as a killer (Winter et al., 2007). For example, another serial killer, John Paul Knowles, described how his new 'career' enabled him to see himself as 'the only successful member of my family' (Wilson & Wilson, 1995, p. 346). A view of oneself as successful and powerful is in marked contrast to the experiences of humiliation that are evident in the histories of many serial killers: for example, as described by one of these, Andrei Chikatilo, who had mutilated and murdered over 50 people, 'It seems that impotence has hounded me all my life. It's ruined my whole life. . . . I felt like a eunuch, humiliated like I wasn't a man at all. Like I was deprived of something basic. All my life, I've felt humiliated' (Cullen, 1999).

For Brady (2001), serial killing may also be a way of attempting to impose some certainty on a chaotic world: the 'serial killer *has* confronted the chaos or absurdity of existence . . . and is trying to impose on it some meaning or order of his own' (p. 102, italics in original). He also viewed it as a choice not 'to exist as a grey daub on a grey canvas' but rather 'as an existential riot of every colour in the spectrum' (p. 82). That Brady had a much more differentiated view of serial killers than of people in general was indicated by a method in which his book was converted to, and analyzed as, a repertory grid, but this also suggested that he tended to dissociate himself from other serial killers.

### Mass murder and terrorism

Before he embarked on a killing spree that left 77, mostly young people attending a Labour Party youth camp, dead, the Norwegian mass murderer Anders Behring Breivik emailed a compendium entitled '2083: A Declaration of European Independence', on which he had worked for some nine years, to over 1,000 addresses. Buried deep within the 1,516 pages of this document is an 'interview with a Justiciar Knight Commander of the PCCTS'[1]. This is essentially an interview with himself, and therefore is not entirely dissimilar to the 'self-characterizations' that Kelly (1955) asked his clients to write and which he used to elucidate their construing (Winter & Tschudi, 2015). It includes a description of various incidents from his early life which might be expected to have shaken his childhood view of the world, or invalidated this view to use the language of personal construct theory. Nevertheless, he considers that he 'had a privileged upbringing with responsible and intelligent people around' him (Berwick, 2011, p. 1387), and he reserves any criticism of this upbringing to the liberal sociopolitical influences to which his family was subjected. His description of his adolescence includes accounts of being a gang member and forming alliances with Muslim gangs, which he admired because of their self-respect and readiness to use violence. However, he then experienced numerous incidents of assaults, threats, abuse and probable humiliation by Muslims. Further apparent invalidation followed in his attempts to embark on political and business careers, but he then 'reestablished' himself as 'A perfect example which should be copied, applauded and celebrated. The Perfect Knight I have always strived to be. A Justiciar Knight is a destroyer of multiculturalism, and as such; a destroyer of evil and a bringer of light' (Berwick, 2011, p. 1435). This included advocating 'armed resistance', involving the deaths of 45,000 and the wounding of a million 'cultural Marxists and multiculturalists'. At the same time, he was able to see himself as 'someone who wouldn't be willing to hurt a fly' (p. 1395), reconciling this inconsistency with the belief that 'In many ways, morality has lost its meaning in our struggle. The question of good and evil is reduced to one simple choice. . . . Survive or perish' (p. 846). The survival for which he saw himself fighting was of Western values in the face of the threat of 'Islamization'.

If Muslim people inconveniently did not behave in a way that validated his view of them as threatening and violent, Breivik considered that they should be incited into doing so. Thus, he stated that 'The most efficient way of infuriating Muslims is to strike at their most prized "possessions", their women. Through deadly and strategic precision attacks (pin prick attacks) we will incite them to engage in violent riots and various forms of Jihadi activities prematurely. The media will have no choice but to cover it, and by doing so contribute to radicalise more Europeans. This spiral will polarise societies and more Europeans will come to learn the "true face of Islam" and multiculturalism.' This is a clear example of the strategy that Kelly (1955) termed hostility, in which one shores up an existing view of the world by extorting evidence for constructions that have been invalidated.

Breivik's story is perhaps not dissimilar to those of many individuals who have found a new structure for their life by becoming radicalized and embarking on a path of terrorism (Winter, 2010). Their lack of compassion for their victims is illustrated by Breivik's statement concerning his stepmother, 'a moderate cultural Marxist and feminist', that 'Although I care for her a great deal, I wouldn't hold it against the [Knights Templar] if she was executed . . .' because she was 'a willing . . . tool for the Multiculturalist Alliance in the indirect genocide of Norwegians through the continued Islamisation of Norway'. It is only when the hardened killer is confronted by the humanity of his or her victims that the full horror of their acts may be felt. For example, as described by a member of a terrorist organization who had committed many acts of violence without remorse but then experienced symptoms of post-traumatic stress disorder after carrying out a shooting:

> he was crying, begging, talking about his children. . . . I was becoming more agitated listening to him, then I looked straight into his face and shot him in the head . . . blood spurted on my suit, he fell, I had to step over him and slipped in the blood and fell on top of him, I panicked and ran.
>
> (Pollock, 2000, p. 179)

### Genocide

Another person who presided over mass murder, in his case of well over a million people, and wrote an autobiographical account (Hoess, 2000), was Rudolf Hoess, the commandant of Auschwitz concentration camp. Using the method of converting his book to a repertory grid that had been used with Ian Brady's book, Hoess was found to view himself as very different from other people but to construe himself as a young man as most similar to Jews (Reed, Winter, Aslan, Soldevilla & Kuzu, 2014). From the perspective of Landfield's (1954) exemplification hypothesis (see Chapter 7), it may be that Jews were threatening to him because they represented an old and rejected part of himself and that this may have contributed to his willingness to play a major part in their extermination. Like Breivik, despite these activities, and despite his acknowledgement that others were likely to perceive him as a 'cruel sadist' and 'bloodthirsty beast', he regarded himself as someone who was 'never cruel', 'had a heart' and was 'not indifferent to human suffering'.

In personal construct theory terms, guilt is the experience of being dislodged from one's core role, the way in which one characteristically sees oneself in relation to others. For Hoess, it was apparent that this core role involved doing his duty and obeying orders, in his case of his superior Heinrich Himmler and ultimately of the Führer. His dedicated and highly efficient implementation of the 'Final Solution' of the 'Jewish problem' therefore caused him no guilt: indeed, quite the reverse. Paradoxically, what did lead him to feel guilty was his awareness not that prisoners had been killed but that they had been mistreated, since this was contrary to orders.

A very similar story is that of Comrade Duch, who commanded S-21, the interrogation centre of the Khmer Rouge in Cambodia, and whose role was to arrange for the extraction of manufactured 'confessions' under torture from prisoners who, if they survived the torture, were then executed. His task was effectively 'to manufacture a new conception of the world' (Panh, 2013, p. 259), and the vigour with which he pursued this was indicated by the fact that of the 14,000 or so prisoners who passed through the gates of S-21, only 7 survived. By organizing torture and death in an orderly, codified fashion, Duch was able to feel pride that 'I applied myself. I never violated discipline' and to believe that 'Malice and cruelty formed no part of our ideology' (Panh, 2013, p. 118). Therefore, like Hoess, his work did not appear to give him cause for guilt, but what did trouble him was learning that orders had been violated in that prisoners had been subjected to forms of torture that (unlike methods such as eating excrement, electrocution of the genitals, and vivisection) were not on an official, prescribed list.

## Pathways to violence

Although every individual's pathway to violence is different, some common features are apparent in the stories presented above.

### Search for meaning

In their various ways, each of these perpetrators of violence found some meaning in their actions, in some cases in contrast to a view of the world that had been subject to persistent invalidation. This new meaning often drew on prevalent social constructions and discourses, for example involving a clear view of a particular group as responsible for invalidation of core aspects of the individual's construing and therefore threatening. If the new view of the world were also invalidated, the individual could always act in such a way as to manufacture evidence in support of it.

### Reconstruction of the self

A similar process to the search for meaning was recovery from experiences such as humiliation, in which there was invalidation of the person's view of the self. The emergence of a new self-construction as a stronger, more powerful, and even heroic person was often achieved by the domination of others or viewing oneself as a saviour of society from some threatening, and perhaps hated, group. Effectively, the individual developed a new 'career' or 'way of life' (Fransella, 1970) which afforded the person more certainty and structure than his or her past self.

### Avoidance of guilt

Acts of violence and terror could be committed without guilt if the individual viewed them as consistent with his or her core role: indeed, not committing such acts against a group perceived as a threat would be a more likely source of guilt. Avoidance of any personal responsibility for acts of violence could also be achieved by the individual viewing himself or herself as only doing his or her duty and obeying orders.

### Dehumanization

Guilt can also be avoided by dehumanizing and depersonalizing one's victims. In the words of Duch, 'Comrades under arrest were enemies, not men' (Panh, 2013, p. 251). Similarly, Nazi propaganda exhorted that the Jews were vermin; while the genocide perpetrated by Hutus in Rwanda was fuelled by radio announcements that their Tutsi victims were 'cockroaches'. In the Vietnam War, US soldiers, referring to the Vietnamese as 'gooks' rather than as people, amused themselves by playing 'gook hockey', in which they gambled on who could hit the most Vietnamese children with their trucks (Appy, 2003). More recently, in the Iraq War, Lieutenant Colonel Fred Swann, who dropped bombs on a restaurant in which Saddam Hussein was reported (wrongly) to be eating, said that 'I did not know who was there. I really didn't care. We've got to get the bombs on target. We've got 10 minutes to do it. We've got to make a lot of things happen to make that happen. So you just fall totally into execute mode and kill the target' (Borger and Millar, 2003). Although the intended target was not killed, many civilians were, but his mechanistic, dehumanized view of his actions and their consequences appeared to allow Swann not to care about this.

## Pathways to violence in the Sierra Leone civil war

As Keen (2005) notes in his analysis of the conflict in Sierra Leone, which attempts to take seriously 'the subjectivity of the violent' (p. 54), 'analysing the causes of violence can seem dangerously close to justifying it' (p. 4). As indicated above, violence of the type that has been described in this book may instead be viewed as incomprehensible, mindless, chaotic and anarchic; or as brutal, evil and beyond the realm of humanity, or at least only characteristic of 'savages' rather than the more refined and developed humans we consider ourselves to be. It bears repetition that, in this way, we are able to distance ourselves from such acts of extreme violence and to avoid the uncomfortable acknowledgement that, as Chandler (2000) remarked in his account of the Khmer Rouge interrogation centre, 'To find the source of the evil that was enacted at S-21 on a daily basis, we need look no further than ourselves.'

To attempt an understanding of the perpetration of extreme violence in the civil war in Sierra Leone, we shall now consider these acts in terms of the pathways to violence delineated above.

### Search for meaning

The discourses of the Revolutionary United Front (RUF) emphasized the grievances of, and deprivation and injustice suffered by, the people of Sierra Leone over the years at the hands of corrupt 'big men' and exploitative foreign powers. This was a situation in which an ordinary person's dreams of success would be likely to be persistently invalidated, and in which RUF propaganda potentially offered an attractive new (albeit perhaps not very coherent) meaning to the lives of many marginalized and disaffected youth.

Even when children and young people did have a clear sense of meaning in their lives, for example in the form of a stable family and community, the rebels often destroyed this meaning by, for example, killing (or forcing children to kill) their families and community members. Young people were also often forced into positions, for example of committing atrocities or being raped, which would have caused them to be ostracized by their communities. They were then ripe for the provision of an alternative identity and meaning, often involving violence, offered by the rebel commanders.

Ian Brady (2001) considered that serial killers, in attempting to impose some order in a chaotic world, can 'often regard destruction as an act of creation' (p. 102). Somewhat similarly, Richards (1996) has described how the actions of the Sierra Leone rebels created in their country 'the wasteland they always supposed it to be' (p. 13). Their actions thus were essentially hostile, in Kelly's (1955) sense, in that they allowed them to extort evidence for their existing views.

## Reconstruction of the self

As Keen (2005) has described, rebel soldiers often moved (or in Kelly's [1955] terms, slot rattled) from a position in which they had felt disempowered, humiliated, shamed and abused to one in which they could view themselves as powerful, for example by humiliating, shaming and abusing others by such acts as mutilation, rape and mockery. In the case of child soldiers, as we have seen in Chapter 5, in so doing, their self-esteem may have been boosted. Such experiences of shame and humiliation were not confined to the rebels, and may have been a factor in the violence that was also perpetrated against civilians by government soldiers, who increasingly felt betrayed and disrespected by the army hierarchy and the government, and some of whom reacted to this by becoming 'sobels'.

For many of these individuals, extreme violence had hardly been unfamiliar before the war, and its use by politicians in Sierra Leone has been seen as leading to a belief 'that violence pays, that it is or can be a way of life, and that it is the shortest and most effective route to achievement and success' (Foray, cited in Keen, 2005). The situation of many young people fighting in the war may therefore have been similar to that of a murderer in a very different setting interviewed by Gresswell and Hollin (1997): 'I've seen violence as a kid (at home, in the street) and I've grown up feeling that violence is a natural thing. I've got a right' (p. 158). For some former child soldiers, an addiction to violence persisted after the war, as in the case of Daniel, whose initiation to violence had involved being forced to amputate the hands of his parents and other family members, who were then shot. After the war, he said that 'to kill, when once you have started, you feel you are highly committed with drugs. It's not drugs. It's the killing. That is the kind of mind you develop' (Bergner, 2005, p. 103).

## Avoidance of guilt

In a morality that had been 'turned on its head' to such an extent that commission of atrocities was rewarded and refusal to commit them punished, guilt for perpetration of violence could easily be avoided in the Sierra Leone conflict by viewing oneself as dutifully obeying orders or following the 'young warrior' role legitimized by secret societies. Responsibility for such actions could also be avoided by attributing them to the effects of drugs or supernatural forces (Keen, 2005).

As Keen (2005) points out, the rebels were not necessarily without moral principles, such as a sense of fairness towards the vulnerable and underprivileged, which might have enabled some of them, like Anders Breivik, to see their actions as committed in the ultimate interests of society. Indeed, the RUF made such statements as 'We are religiously godly in our bearings and beliefs', as well as 'We have learnt the value of treating captives and prisoners of war with utmost civility' (Revolutionary United Front, 1995). This may be no more easy to accept than Ian Brady's (2001) statement that 'Serial killers, like it or not, can possess just as many admirable facets of character as anyone else, and sometimes more than average. . . . They also have their own personal code of ethics and morals, albeit eccentric to the ordinary individual'. However, the point is that it is transgression of the individual's own personal moral code that will elicit guilt, and in the case of a rebel soldier or a serial killer this code may be very different from that of most people.

### Dehumanization

No less than in other wars, combatants in Sierra Leone dehumanized their victims, the rebels making statements such as 'the civilian has no blood' (Muana, 1997, p. 80). Drug taking appeared to facilitate this process, with reports by rebel soldiers that drug use made them seem very tall and civilians as small as insects (Keen, 2005). This was sometimes coupled with a certain dehumanization of themselves, but seeing the self as a fierce animal such as a tiger or cobra rather than vermin like their victims.

## Conclusions

Rather than being incomprehensible, acts of extreme violence can be viewed in terms of 'normal' psychological processes such as a search for meaning and the reconstruction of the self following persistent invalidation. These processes may be coupled with a 'hostile' extortion of evidence for the individual's view of the world; avoidance of guilt; and dehumanization of victims of violence. Analysis in these terms may be applied to individuals who engage in serial or mass killing but also to soldiers who commit atrocities in warfare throughout the world, including the conflict in Sierra Leone. It, of course, focuses on the individual psychological, rather than broader systemic or political, roots of violence. However, arguably it may lead to greater possibilities for prevention of violence, by taking seriously the search for meaning that may underlie it and attempting to reconstruct a new meaning that does not involve violence, than dismissing violent acts as evil or insane.

## Note

1  Pauperes commilitones Christi Templique Solomonici (the Poor Fellow-Soldiers of Christ and of the Temple of Solomon).

## References

Appy, C. G. (2003) *Vietnam: The definitive oral history told from all sides.* London: Ebury Press.
Bergner, D. (2005) *Soldiers of light.* London: Penguin Books.

Berwick, A. (2011) *2083: A European declaration of independence.* Available at: http://www.slideshare.net/darkandgreen/2083-a-european-declaration-of-independence-by-andrew-berwick [Accessed 28 July 2011].

Borger, J., Millar, S. (2003, 9 April) Countdown: How technology helped pinpoint Iraqi leader. *The Guardian.*

Brady, I. (2001) *The gates of Janus: Serial killing and its analysis.* Los Angeles: Feral House.

Chandler, D. (2000) *Voices from S-21.* Chiang Mai, Thailand: Silkworm.

Cullen, R. (1999) *The killer department.* London: Orion.

Fransella, F. (1970) Stuttering: Not a symptom but a way of life. *British Journal of Communication Disorders,* 5: 22–29.

Gresswell, D. M., Hollin, C. R. (1997) Addictions and multiple murder: A behavioural perspective. In J. E. Hodge, M. McMurran, C. R. Hollin (Eds.), *Addicted to crime?* (pp. 139–164). Chichester: Wiley.

Hoess, R. (2000) *Commandant of Auschwitz.* London: Phoenix Press.

Horley, J. (Ed.) (2003) *Personal construct perspectives on forensic psychology.* London: Routledge.

Houston, J. (1998) *Making sense with offenders: Personal constructs, therapy and change.* Chichester: Wiley.

Keen, D. (2005) *Conflict and collusion in Sierra Leone.* Oxford: James Currey.

Kelly, G. A. (1955) *The psychology of personal constructs.* New York: Norton. (Reprinted by Routledge, 1991)

Landfield, A. W. (1954) A movement interpretation of threat. *Journal of Abnormal and Social Psychology,* 49: 529–532.

Muana, P. K. (1997) The Kamajoi militia: Violence, internal displacement and the politics of counter-insurgency. *Africa Development,* XXII, 77–100.

Panh, R. (2013) *The elimination: A survivor of the Khmer Rouge confronts his past and the commandant of the killing fields.* London: Clerkenwell Press.

Pollock, P. H. (2000) Eye movement desensitization and reprocessing (EMDR) for post-traumatic stress disorder (PTSD) following homicide. *Journal of Forensic Psychiatry,* 11: 176–184.

Reed, N., Winter, D., Aslan, E., Soldevilla, J. M., Kuzu, D. (2014) An exemplary life? A personal construct analysis of the autobiography of Rudolf Hoess, commandant of Auschwitz. *Journal of Constructivist Psychology,* 27: 274–288.

Revolutionary United Front (1995) *Footpaths to democracy: Toward a new Sierra Leone.* Available at: http://www.sierra-leone.org/AFRC-RUF/footpaths.html [Accessed 5 August 2015].

Richards, P. (1996) *Violence as cultural creativity: Social exclusion and environmental damage in Sierra Leone.* Mimeo.

Wilson, C., Wilson, D. (1995) *A plague of murder: The rise and rise of serial killing in the modern age.* London: Robinson.

Winter, D. A. (2007) Construing the construction processes of serial killers and violent offenders: 2. The limits of credulity. *Journal of Constructivist Psychology,* 20: 247–275.

Winter, D. A. (2010) Radicalisation as a constructive choice: Possible research directions. In S. Sassaroli, G. Ruggiero, Y. Ergas (Eds.), *Perspectives on immigration and terrorism* (pp. 115–119). Amsterdam: IOS Press.

Winter, D. A., Feixas, G., Dalton, R., Jarque-Llamazares, L., Laso, E., Mallindine, C., Patient, S. (2007) Construing the construction processes of serial killers and violent offenders: 1. The analysis of narratives. *Journal of Constructivist Psychology,* 20: 1–22.

Winter, D., Tschudi, F. (2015) Construing a 'perfect knight': A personal construct investigation of mass murder. *Journal of Constructivist Psychology,* 28: 139–151.

# Chapter 13

# Forgiveness and reconciliation

How can survivors of conflict transition from a state of war to good reintegration, coming back together as communities of belonging once again? Forgiveness, foundational for a good life, is essential for this task, as it has direct bearing on the existence and quality of relationships between people (Willmer, 2003; Wright, 1996). Additionally, it is believed to have direct bearing on one's well-being (Cohen, 2004); without it, peace of mind and agency are challenged (Care, 2002).

Discussions about forgiveness can be found throughout various disciplines and considered in light of its cultural, political, spiritual and collective context.[1] As could be expected, there are similarities and differences, both in philosophy and practical approach. In the Sierra Leonean context, how is forgiveness understood? How do culture, religion and politics influence forgiveness, both in understanding and in its enactment? Forgiveness may involve from one to multiple parties to the offence; an intrapersonal approach to the interpersonal and communal approach. What is the significance of community in the forgiveness process, which then has direct bearing on reintegration and recovery?

Some offences are regarded more seriously depending on the cultural context. Does this have a bearing on forgiveness, thus making some offences appear more 'justifiably' forgivable than others? Would it be easier to invoke the 'forgive and forget' approach that seems so needed in situations of extreme violence if the victim were to avoid the offender or the offender to deny that offences have been committed? Yet it is doubtful this would work; public life demands that we choose whether or not to forgive (Arendt, 1958). This is particularly the case in the long run and in the context of a war-torn society. A huge tub of molasses, called 'Avoidance and Denial', will hide the table tennis ball called 'Offence' when pushed underneath the surface. However, its disappearance is temporary. It will resurface!

Forgiveness is language, but it is also and essentially action. What does this look like? Additionally, how does forgiving and receiving forgiveness support agency and resilience, the capacity not only to survive but also to overcome and even flourish despite or even as a result of the difficulties that have severely challenged them? These questions highlight some of the issues we will consider in this chapter, which draws upon the stories of war survivors and considers the extent to which forgiveness is possible.

## Cultural constructs and expressions of the language of forgiveness

We begin with an examination of the cultural constructs and expressions of the language of forgiveness found within Sierra Leone. Forgiveness language is not foreign to Sierra Leone. The Sierra Leonean population is a mix of Muslim, Christian, and traditional religions, some practising all three (Goins, 2015). This is not unusual for African society (Rieber, 1977).

President Kabbah, in 26 of his speeches addressing the nation, parliament and various organizations, refers to forgiving, in the metaphor of embrace, as is exemplified below:

> In my first year in office . . . I . . . embark(ed) upon a course of reconciliation, the healing of wounds and closing of the rifts that had existed within our society. . . . I treated the misdemeanours and misdeeds of certain people with compassion and a spirit of forgiveness. With open arms, I welcomed them like prodigal sons who had left the shores of Sierra Leone, perhaps for good, and others who were forced into exile.
>
> (Kabbah, 1998)[2]

Kabbah urged victims of the war '. . . to forgive the perpetrators of the atrocities committed against them. I am convinced that with a successful disarmament it is only by such acts of forgiveness and reconciliation that lasting peace can return to Sierra Leone' (Kabbah, 2000). He stated his commitment to the proper investigation of human rights abuses, supported by the United Nations and the Lomé Peace Agreement. Clearly, one goal was reconciliation through forgiveness (Goins, 2015).

There were examples of similar requests. Sankoh and Koroma urged their own followers in like manner, addressing approximately 800 former soldiers and hundreds of local residents and asking the civilian population's forgiveness of former soldiers. RUF leader Colonel Mohamed Kallon apologized to ECOMOG, UNAMSIL and AFRC officials and asked forgiveness for abuses perpetrated against the civilian population. 'The meeting concluded with a friendly football game between the Port Loko team and that of Lunsar',[3] indicating their intentions to let the past be the past.

Despite ongoing violations from the RUF and AFRC, President Kabbah continued his appeal to the population to forgive. Many children said, '*The government said we should forgive*', when they spoke of atrocities they personally experienced from the rebels, some of the rebels being children themselves. One 14-year-old child wrote, '*Now when the war finished, they announced it every day and night that people should forgive the rebels so that Sierra Leone will have peace*' (Goins, 2015).

Interviewees affirmed this. A journalist who travelled with Kabbah from October 1999 until May 2001 said, '*At every stop he told people that if former fighters came to them and sincerely asked their forgiveness, then they should forgive them*'.[4] Momoh, a youth who cofounded the Community Theatre Agency, which will be discussed later in this chapter, witnessed this, and also participated in one of Kabbah's presentations calling for reintegration of former soldiers, adults and children.

Forgiveness language from these political figures could be understood as forbearance of revenge (Shriver, 1995); political acts of apology rather than personal repentance (Biggar, 2001); or, directed forgiveness where people are required to forgive (Govier, 2006). Even though the state must work towards societal and political restoration, Govier contends that this way of doing so puts undue and unfair pressure on victims. Van Deusen Hunsinger (2001, p. 91) says demanding forgiveness 'can be a form of moral violence'.

The Inter-Religious Council of Sierra Leone (IRCSL) was a proactive advisory body to President Kabbah. They represented the attitudes of religious leaders and followers at a crucial point in Sierra Leonean history. According to interviewees, the actions of the IRCSL modelled constructs of forgiveness through their participation in the Truth and Reconciliation Commission (TRC), to be discussed later. Additionally, they influenced civil society groups to initiate practices of forgiveness through reintegration and reconciliation, such as the Council of Churches, and were actively preaching forgiveness in both churches and mosques (Goins, 2015).

The IRCSL had a substantial role in forming the Lomé Peace Agreement. They were the first 'to move into the jungle to preach the message of peace to the rebels' (Karimu, 2001) and to pray for 'resistant hard liners' (Turay, 2000, p. 53). Fornah Usman, a minister and IRCSL member, said the following:

> We are always preaching the ministry of reconciliation. No matter what those guys may have done, there is room on the side of the Lord to forgive them and to bring them back on the road they are supposed to be on.
>
> (Turay, 2000, p. 53)

Civil society and government respected the IRCSL for speaking out for 'repentance, forgiveness and reconciliation' (Turay, 2000). They met with paramount chiefs and traditional leaders, UN officials and their constituencies, facilitating training in community-based reconciliation, rituals and cleansing ceremonies (Mundy, 2005, p. 50).

Thus, within the cultural context of Sierra Leone, forgiveness language proved to be useful for transitioning from war to peaceful coexistence. As Montville (1993, p. 124) notes, if 15 to 20 per cent of the population takes on a change of attitude towards the enemy, 'it takes on a diffusion rate that cannot be stopped'. Therefore, consistent messages to forgive coming from the state were justified, and certainly influenced other reintegration efforts by INGOs, NGOs and the civilian population (Goins, 2015).

### 'Forgive and forget' and 'ow for do'

'Forgive and forget' and 'ow for do' are common expressions associated with the forgiveness and reconciliation process post-war. These expressions make reference to different ways of 'forgiving' acknowledged as useful by Sierra Leoneans.

To forgive and forget is to acknowledge and move on, to not bear a grudge (Goins, 2015). According to some Sierra Leoneans, this way of forgiving made reintegration and reconciliation possible. It was a way of remembering – not forgetting – by not allowing past memories to poison the present and future, or as Shaw (2004b) noted, not giving them a strong voice.

By promising conditional amnesty to the former opposition soldiers, President Kabbah encouraged forgiving and a kind of forgetting. As people saw positive some developments after the war, they were able to move past the atrocities (Keen, 2005). For instance, one interviewee (#26) spoke about youth having a youth minister post-war and females going to school.

'I will forgive but I will not forget' was by far the most common arrangement of the two words post-war. As one person (Interviewee #7) reflected, *'You can forgive somebody but it is very difficult to forget. . . . You will forgive, but if you see something like that again, your mind will reflect back to what has happened to you before.'* In other words, the incident is put aside for practical purposes more than anything else. Feelings have changed, as Interviewee #13 said: *'I'm sorry it happened because we cannot have the same love.'* Unfortunately, people who forgive but do not forget may be captured by the memory and pain of the offence. 'You don't really forgive, you don't really forget. You simply accept that there's nothing you can do to change what has happened' (Jackson, 2004, p. 68).

This is the basic meaning behind 'ow for do', which means 'what can be done' or 'there is nothing left to do'. One has to move on. It is also an expression reflecting a fatalistic culture. Whether that 'moving on' is a sort of resignation or a determination to take action will be the critical determinant for forgiveness and reconciliation.

To forgive but purposely not forget can have another meaning, useful to society and to talk about forgiveness. Several interviewees expressed the importance of not forgetting:

> *We don't want to forget. . . . We owe it to our children not to forget . . . and to address the causes. This is the reason for not forgetting. . . . That's why we have to be reminded of the causes of this catastrophe.*
>
> (Interviewee #27)

This posture towards forgetting is consistent with some reactions to horrendous events such as the Rwandan genocide, the Holocaust, or the Apartheid system and rule in South Africa. Memorials erected, specific days in history commemorated and 'nationalized', and rituals and traditions enshrined within a community all speak to the actions of purposely remembering so as not to forget. 'Remember and forgive . . . (R)emember in such a way . . . as to drain the memory of its power to continue to poison the present and future' (Shriver, 2003, p. 31).

## Seeing and enacting forgiveness

### Rebuilding community: the Community Theatre Agency

One of the most innovative efforts to foster forgiveness and reconciliation was through the Community Theatre Agency (CTA), a grassroots effort founded by Momoh and his friends who fought with him in their village civil defence force (CDF). While Momoh and his friends were fighting with the CDF, some of their other village friends had been abducted by the RUF. Momoh found himself fighting against these (RUF) friends. When the war was over, reintegration for him was a given; however, his friends in the RUF were not welcomed back into their village. Theirs was not a unique situation. What they learnt in their own community, they continued to employ in other villages following protocol to ensure that they would be welcomed by chiefs and elders.

In order to see a community restored, Momoh and his CDF friends (a group of eight) spent time amongst the people assessing how to promote reconciliation with former RUF soldiers. They conducted 'listening surveys', identifying obstacles to reintegration. Having gathered enough relevant information, they presented what they had learnt and possible solutions through dramatic skits.

> We presented what the rebels did, because you can't beg for forgiveness if you don't identify the problem. . . . Even in the sketch you see the rebel coming into the community, with that sign of remorse. Because that is the questions they (the community) are asking, 'will the rebels show a sign of remorse, that they are sorry about it?' It is very, very, very important, if you don't show remorse. Nobody will appreciate you are sorry if you don't do it right.

Performances were no more than 30 minutes, with skits and then singing. Afterwards, . . .

> We ask them . . . what do you understand from it? Some say it tells us how to forgive the rebels that are in the bush so that we can live together; some will say we have to embrace our brothers that are coming back from the bush; some will say we have to have peace. We ask them, is it really proper that our brothers − normally, we don't call them rebels, we call them brothers so they themselves know they are part of one family. So we say, is it possible for our brothers who are in the bush to stay there or to come back? And they say, we want them to come.
>
> So from there we start killing that spirit of violence. . . . They will end up saying, there is nothing we can do, we have to accept them. That is the way we are using the play, in order to kill the spirit of violence and take up the spirit of acceptance.

Before the skits, Momoh said that villagers would refer to the rebels as just that – rebels.

> *After the acting, you know there is transformation when they won't call them rebels again. They would say, 'These people are our brothers'. So we look for the key points – did the message reach the people. Because in the initial stage, they call them rebels. If they still are calling them rebels, they are not willing to accept them. So then when they are willing to accept them, they call them 'our brothers'.*

The CTA members concluded that when they heard this transition, their message of reconciliation had penetrated the minds of the villagers.[5]

The CTA did not stop with efforts inside villages, but also initiated reintegration efforts with former soldiers by going to the demobilization camps. In the first camp experience, they interviewed rebels and then did a drama that depicted the actions of the rebels during the war.

> *(B)ut they don't want to see what they've done. A few of them, when we started to act the play, were throwing things at us, chairs, anything they could get. So that day we had to stop because the rebels said we were trying to provoke them. . . . So after . . . the skit, they said, 'We have to acknowledge it. This is what we have done. Now we know what you (the community representatives) are yearning towards us. This is what we have done, and we have to acknowledge it.' . . . . Most times, when we are going to do the play for the rebels, there are some that are very negative. But there are some that are more intelligent. They will listen. At the end of the day . . . they realized they've wronged the society and need to show a sign of remorse when they go back to the society.*

How did Momoh determine that CTA efforts actually made a difference? Their main objective was to rebuild a sense of community and community values. Their own village was a splintered one, with some wanting former soldiers back, while others did not. Some former soldiers longed for acceptance and recognized their need for forgiveness. Others preferred to live apart. At the same time, former soldiers needed to demonstrate a remorseful, repentant attitude to community members who were rightfully very fearful and untrusting. According to Momoh, when CTA members would return to a village in a month or two and see the former rebels walking around, being acknowledged as 'brothers' and 'sisters' by the villagers, they knew their efforts had not been in vain.

### Rebuilding community: as seen in civil society

In children's written discourse, there was example after example of former child soldiers being reintegrated into their families and communities. Only 1 of the 232 former child soldiers who wrote narratives mentioned being rejected by a family member, whom he said 'did not like him'. Otherwise, the only circumstance that altered any of these children living with their parents or family was if they were orphaned during the war (Goins, 2015).

> *After the rebel war, the rebels come to beg for forgiveness so we accept them as our brother and sister, we forgive, we forget about the past, we are [sharing] things in common, we eat together we also look to their [good].*
>
> (#1, a 12-year-old male former soldier)

Adult interviewees confirmed the importance of community rebuilding. They actually took in children whom they knew to have been part of the rebel faction. Interviewees knew of others housing and caring for former child soldiers.

Various organizations made specific efforts to rebuild community, such as the International Committee of the Red Cross (ICRC). The ICRC initiated the Child Advocacy and Rehabilitation Programme (CAR), which identified hindrances to reintegration for former child soldiers. This was for children who did not integrate into the community or were living within a community but as ostracized members. Other organizations sponsored houses for female former soldiers with 'bush babies' who were unable to integrate due to their being stigmatized.

Church leaders and members came together to rebuild community through production of a booklet (Salia, 2000, p. 13).[6] The poem below illustrates the content of the booklet:

> Come home, brothers and sisters
> We are tired of war
> Of its horrifying scenes
> Of rape
> Of maiming and killing
> In blazing towns and villages
> Come home
> Come home to rebuild
> Come home
> Come home to rebuild

One amputee emphasized the importance of rebuilding community in a very practical way. He said of the rebels, 'Let them come out of the bush. I will receive them and we will eat together . . . if we don't forgive they will never leave the bush and the atrocities will continue . . . who will help me then?' (Limbs of Hope, 2001, p. 19).

Some females at the IDP camp experienced quite the opposite. They were pointed at and called rebels by others. Returning to their communities of origin was not even a consideration for them. They remained in the IDP camp living under deplorable conditions and barely able to survive on the monthly allotment of oil and bulgur wheat. While their choice was an alternative to reintegration, it also suggests the importance of community building in their integration. They shared stories and knew one another's past involvement with the RUF. They demonstrated acceptance and mutual forgiveness through their attitudes and conversations. Rather than being rejected outside the IDP camp, they formed their own community and a place of belonging within the camp.

### Rebuilding community: as seen through government

Reintegration and reconciliation between government and armed groups were to begin with a commitment to cease physical violence, the goal being to restore cooperative working relationships and trust between parties. President Kabbah promoted community rebuilding through reintegration while negotiations were taking place between the government and armed groups. Kabbah stated the following in April 1996:

> My government is prepared to give a general amnesty to all members of the RUF in the name of peace. . . . We will also reintegrate these combatants into our society. . . .
>
> (Gberie, 2000, p. 22)

The commitment to amnesty for all former soldiers carried over into the 1999 Lomé Peace Agreement.[7] Through the promise of amnesty, there was a kind of forgiving sanctioned at the political/government level. Perpetrators would not be held legally responsible for their wrongful acts under the condition that they not violate the agreement. Through government-sanctioned reintegration, it was hoped that society would take former soldiers back into the community, which was one of the goals of amnesty (Forsberg, 2003, p. 69). Still, 'the road to peace was to be long and tortuous', as could be expected (Bright, 2000).

The Truth and Reconciliation Commission (TRC) was established '. . . in the spirit of national reconciliation' in order to 'provide a forum for both the victims and perpetrators of human rights violations to tell their story, get a clear picture of the past in order to facilitate genuine healing and reconciliation'.[8] Truth telling was central to the successful functioning of the TRC, as its purpose was to rebuild community in this way. This will be discussed later in the chapter.

The policy of the Ministry of Education was to provide equal education opportunities for all children without discriminating as to whether they were former child soldiers. This open policy represented an act of reconciliation as it promoted reintegration of former child soldiers into the school system. Protecting the identity of the child was technically a priority, though people said everyone knew who they were. The supervisor for the Ministry of Education believed forgiveness was critical to societal reintegration, and believed children needed to learn about forgiveness and its application (Goins, 2015).

While government can inspire and influence civil society, it is only effective insofar as the civil society responds accordingly. Government can encourage and support the rebuilding of community and community values, but it is the people who must do it; it is civil society members who must finally choose to enact interpersonal forgiving.

## Rebuilding community: as seen through social and spiritual transition

Formal and informal practices enable transition from one social state to another, which is relevant to victim and perpetrator, to individuals and to the group. These practices, drawing from culturally relevant customs and concepts, also facilitate the forgiveness process between these groupings of people.

In churches and mosques, religious leaders encouraged reconciliation between former soldiers and community members. In villages, elders and leaders would often do the same. Reconciliation was most successfully facilitated through integration of traditional practices, such as relevant ceremonies or rituals, which are understood to support good reintegration (Baker & May, 2004; Goins, 2015; Krech, 2003; Williamson & Cripe, 2002). Ceremonies and rituals signify a transition from one social state to another for former soldiers (Goins, 2015), from a guilty to a non-guilty state. In the case of Sierra Leone, ceremonies and rituals were often created for the sake of the reintegration process.

Ceremonies and rituals are central to processes of social recovery and community transformation (Goins, 2015; Mundy, 2005). All non-government armed groups initiated their recruits, purportedly imbuing them with magical powers. Even when no longer with the armed group, former soldiers were still mobilized in their minds. A de-initiation process was a critical step towards transformation (Gbla, 2003a; Krech, 2003; Mundy, 2005; Shaw, 2004a).

There is an adage in Sierra Leone that 'there is no bad bush to throw away a bad child' (Gbla, 2003a, p. 188). Enacting traditional rituals reinforces this belief. Several interviewees, as well as NGO staff, noted that in the absence of rituals, reintegration and/or reconciliation is often difficult at best and impossible at worst (Goins, 2015). The IRCSL was active in promoting reintegration of former child soldiers through ceremonies (Mundy, 2005). Shaw (2004a) speaks of adult family members rubbing blessed water on children and 'transforming' their hearts from fighters into children. Rituals thus reconnected children with their communities. Williamson and Cripe (2002) noted that for females, traditional ceremonies and rituals are believed to cleanse them from the violence done against them and assist in their psychological healing.

Rituals and ceremonies '. . . appease the spirits of the dead in order to save both the perpetrators and their communities from the wrath of these spirits' (Gbla, 2003a, p. 187). Gbla advocates for traditional healers and local artisans in the rehabilitation and reintegration process. Some noted that Christian doctrine was compatible with the traditional practices of local healers.[9]

The NCDDR also utilized rituals and ceremonies for reintegration and reconciliation. In one such ceremony, a former RUF commander was questioned about his commitment to a nonviolent lifestyle. He was asked to declare his intentions to be arms-free to the questioning UNAMSIL commander, who then guided him to go down on his knees. The former RUF commander was surrounded by other UNAMSIL soldiers. He began destroying his AK-47 with various tools, which was meant to demonstrate his commitment to peace. He was then asked, 'Now that you are a civilian, what do you intend to do?' He replied, 'Go back and help develop Sierra Leone.' Soldiers formerly under his command went through the same procedure.[10]

Onlookers were asked how they felt about these former soldiers returning to their areas, before and after the ceremonies. Before the disarming and accompanying ceremonies, civilians said they were afraid. However, after the disarming and ceremonies, they were not. Undoubtedly, attitudinal transformation takes more time. However, perhaps seeing the NCDDR's efforts in combination with the desire for a new start all worked to make the ceremonies effective for reintegrating purposes.

Gbla (2003a) cites an incident in which a 15-year-old boy, conscripted by the RUF, returned to his village. Upon his return, the family and village elders put him in a grass hut to be used for his cleansing ceremony. Inside, the boy removed clothing worn while he was with the RUF. After setting fire to the hut, an adult relative helped the boy to escape. The burning ritual signified the boy's break with the 'evil past'. To bring peace to the boy and community, a chicken was sacrificed. Voeten (2000) describes a similar kind of cleansing ceremony. After the high priest fasts for 10 days, he takes the child – dressed in old clothes – and parents to a hut and 'prays to the spirits of the ancestors, asking them for forgiveness. The child is washed with the sacred water and dressed in clean clothes' (Voeten, 2000, p. 247). Following the ceremony, the village receives the 'new' child.

Oftentimes, children are reintegrated into their communities without ceremony.[11] Reintegrated children, particularly girls, wrote about being raped but did not speak of an accompanying ceremony (Goins, 2015). Still, rituals and ceremonies are significant in the reintegration process for former child soldiers. Enactments of forgiveness are featured in interpersonal, collective and spiritual dimensions, within the traditional practices of rituals and ceremonies that incorporate signs of repentance.

### Rebuilding community: the Truth and Reconciliation Commission

The TRC was critical to facilitating an exchange between perpetrator and victim and, through chiefs, religious leaders and relevant ceremonies, reintegrating former combatants into their home communities (Lorey & Beezley, 2002, p. 253). People had opportunities to relay their personal stories at the public hearings and through the statement-taking process. Sessions began with a time for victims and perpetrators to give their testimonies (TRC, 2004). People could listen to the sessions on the radio if they were not able to be present (Goins, 2015). Perpetrators in particular were severely questioned by the residing, usually local, officials. At the conclusion of the hearing, perpetrators could publicly apologize and be officially exonerated by the ceremony officiator, be that priest, elder or chief (Goins, 2015; TRC, 2004).

Thus, the TRC provided a forum for perpetrator and victim '. . . to be healed, . . . to reconcile with self . . . and neighbour(s) and . . . community, . . . to be reunited, . . . reintegrated, to help repair . . . shattered . . . communities' (Kelsall, 2004). The narratives below from two interviewees (#19 and #26, in Goins, 2015) provide examples of the TRC protocol:

> *The TRC would be at the community and then the person would . . . tell how he was abducted and what the rebels had done to him, and then he would apologize. The TRC would hand him over to the chief and the elders, . . . and they would listen to his apologies and then the chief would be called on to talk, and he would say, 'You are our child and we take you back into our society, into our community. Let us see how we can rebuild Sierra Leone'.*
>
> *They use to come and say, 'You have killed my father at so and so time, on so and so day, and I know that you are the one. But I have forgiven you'. . . . So it just came out naturally. People started accepting one another, people that killed the relative of somebody would come and say, 'It's me that killed your relative'. (The victim would say) 'I have forgiven you'. (The perpetrator would say) 'Have mercy on me'.*

This interviewee said, '*So people were going around to reconcile with one another. Because it is the only option. We are living in community.*' In other words, living in community is the only reasonable and viable option for Sierra Leoneans. Another interviewee (#24) said perpetrators '*were testifying with tears so you could see the guilt feelings come out*'. For the most part, the TRC was seen to be helpful in the transition and reintegration process, '*a step in the right direction*'.[12]

Interestingly, the TRC did not hold anyone under 12 as responsible or accountable for their actions as soldiers, which some believed was a mistake, particularly if the child had been a commando. '*You are a responsible somebody if you are in charge of some other people.*'[13] Therefore, the TRC was not helpful in their reintegration because it did not make a place for their transitioning.

According to Shaw (2004b), the TRC may have disrupted local communities' practices of reintegration and reconciliation. In order to protect their communities and relationships, an entire community would agree to withhold information potentially damaging to the families of former soldiers. Thus, communities demonstrated a forgiving attitude towards former soldiers through a lack of cooperation with the TRC. Nevertheless, within the TRC proceedings, forgiveness, enacted invitationally, bilaterally and collectively, supported reintegration.

### Rebuilding community: story telling and tradition

Story telling and traditional songs and games are useful in constructing 'new identities' for youth (Mundy, 2005). Story telling served as a transitioning element for former child soldiers within the practices of the TRC, in part because it is integral to Sierra Leonean culture. It is an indirect approach to problem solving or as a means of saving face (Abu-Nimer, 2003; Elmer, 1993). Despite the brutality of their stories, most people were eager to talk (Goins, 2015). Hearing the 'real' stories of former soldiers helped listeners think about them differently.

'Our history tells us to tell our stories,' one IDP female said (Goins, 2015). Story telling serves two purposes here. First, there is the chance for psychosocial healing that comes with the belief that one is not being judged but rather understood. Second, sharing one's story offers the possibility to move beyond the old story to a new and different story. Sorie's (referenced in Chapter 5) desire to bring everything out in the open overrode his natural inclination to 'cover up' shameful acts. He wanted, more, a new story, rather than live in bondage to his old story. Story telling facilitated repentance and self-forgiveness (Goins, 2015).

Limbs of Hope (LOH) researchers noted that amputee victims, as they shared their stories, experienced a positive transition in their emotional responses to the trauma they had experienced during and after the amputation. Reportedly, their strong negative emotions subsided in the recounting. Though they were not afforded the opportunity to confront the perpetrator, the change in attitude suggests unilateral forgiving. For these and other victims whose perpetrators were unknown, a new story might only come through this kind of forgiving (Goins, 2015).

## Conclusions

In this chapter, we have recounted how reintegration of former soldiers is based on enacted constructs of forgiveness. The field data illustrated the obvious benefits to forgiveness and suggested methods for realizing forgiveness, both involving reintegration. Thus, community is significant in the process of forgiveness.

In fact, forgiveness 'is essential to every society and all politics. . . . Without some mechanism for letting go (forgiving) of old grievances, every set of relationships, whether a marriage, a community, or a nation, will eventually collapse or explode.' Forgiveness and repentance 'offer the possibility of injecting a fresh impulse into a situation characterized by automatic reaction' (Liechty, 1998, p. 173). Beginning anew is impossible when, as Wright (1998) notes, relationships are characterized by old fears and histories and vulnerabilities. Forgiveness and repentance can symbolize the new and offer individuals, communities and societies a way to begin anew.

## Notes

1  See the following sources: Biggar, 2001; Gbla, 2003b; Jones, 1995; Murphy & Hampton, 1988; Shriver, 1995; Volf, 1996; Worthington Jr, 1998, 2005.
2  From a speech Kabbah delivered in Freetown's city stadium. Available at: http://www.sierra-leone.org/Speeches/kabbah-031098.html [Accessed 5 August 2015].
3  From *Sierra Leone News*, October 1999. Available at: http://www.sierra-leone.org/Archives/slnews1099.html [Accessed 05 August 2015].
4  Requested to remain anonymous.
5  Interestingly, in several narratives children referred to the former rebels as brothers, their language suggesting an acceptance of them as family.
6  In an effort to contribute to national reconciliation, the Council of Churches in Sierra Leone (CCSL), whose membership represents numerous Christian denominations, published a booklet called *Friends Again* (Salia, 2000). It contains a collection of songs, verses, letters, short plays and prayers for reconciliation penned by various Sierra Leoneans, and was distributed primarily through local churches in the four main regions of Sierra Leone (Bo, Kenema, Makeni and Freetown).
7  The Lomé Peace Agreement was a significant effort from government and armed groups to reestablish peace and security and facilitate a workable reintegration and reconciliation between opposing parties.
8  See Appendix, Article XXVI of the Lomé Peace Agreement.
9  Data from interviewees and narratives affirmed this. Also, see Geschiere (1999).
10  This information is from a CD obtained through someone living in the Makeni District. It is an amateur video, showing a ceremony that occurred in 1998, and has no identifying information on it, such as speakers, producers, etc. Most of the language spoken was Creole.
11  Interviewee #29, whose daughter disappeared for more than a year and was found in a nearby village. The girl did not make any effort to get back to her family on her own.
12  Interviewee #16.
13  Ibid.

## References

Abu-Nimer, M. (2003) *Nonviolence and peace building in Islam: Theory and practice.* Gainesville: University Press of Florida.

Arendt, H. (1958) *The human condition.* Chicago: University of Chicago Press.

Baker, B., May, R. (2004) Reconstructing Sierra Leone. *Commonwealth & Comparative Politics,* 42(1): 35–60.

Biggar, N. (2001) Forgiveness in the twentieth century: A review of the literature, 1901–2001. In A. McFadyen, M. Sarot (Eds.), *Forgiveness and truth* (pp. 181–217). Edinburgh: T & T Clark.

Bright, D. (2000) Implementing the Lomé Peace Agreement. In D. Lord (Ed.), *Paying the price: The Sierra Leonean peace process* (Vol. 9, pp. 36–41). London: Conciliation Resources.

Care, N. S. (2002) Forgiveness and effective agency. In S. Lamb, J. G. Murphy (Eds.), *Before forgiving: Cautionary views of forgiveness in psychotherapy* (pp. 215–231). Oxford: Oxford University Press.

Cohen, A. (2004) *Forgiveness, peace and well-being.* Available at: http://greatergood.berkeley.edu/article/item/the_science_of_forgiveness_an_annotated_bibliography [Accessed 5 August 2015].

Elmer, D. (1993) *Cross-cultural conflict: Building relationships for effective ministry.* Downers Grove, IL: Intervarsity Press.

Forsberg, T. (2003) The philosophy and practice of dealing with the past: Some conceptual and normative issues. In N. Biggar (Ed.), *Burying the past: Making peace and doing justice after civil conflict* (2nd ed., pp. 65–86). Washington, DC: Georgetown University Press.

Gberie, L. (2000) First stages on the road to peace: The Abidjan process. In D. Lord (Ed.), *Paying the price: The Sierra Leonean peace process* (Vol. 9, pp. 18–25). London: Conciliation Sources.

Gbla, O. (2003a) Conflict and post-war trauma among child soldiers in Liberia and Sierra Leone. In A. Sesay (Ed.), *Civil wars, child soldiers and post conflict peace building in West Africa* (pp. 167–194). Ibadan, Nigeria: Nigerian College Press Publishers.

Gbla, O. (2003b) Post-war reconstruction in Liberia and Sierra Leone. In A. Sesay (Ed.), *Civil wars, child soldiers and post conflict peace building in West Africa* (pp. 195–212). Ibadan, Nigeria: Nigeria College Press Publishers.

Geschiere, P. (1999) Globalization and the power of indeterminate meaning: Witchcraft and spirit cults in Africa and East Asia. In B. Meyer, P. Geschiere (Eds.), *Globalization and identity: Dialectics of flow and closure* (pp. 211–237). Oxford: Blackwell.

Goins, S. (2015) *Forgiveness and reintegration: How the transformative process of forgiveness impacts child soldier reintegration* (provisional title). Oxford: Regnum Books.

Govier, T. (2006) *Taking wrongs seriously: Acknowledgment, reconciliation, and the politics of sustainable peace.* Amherst, NY: Humanity Books.

Jackson, M. (2004) *In Sierra Leone.* Durham, NC: Duke University Press.

Jones, G. (1995) *Embodying forgiveness.* Grand Rapids: Eerdmans Publishing Co.

Kabbah, President A.A.T. (1998) *Address to the Nation: 10 March 1998.* Available at: http://www.sierra-leone.org/Speeches/kabbah-031098.html [Accessed 5 August 2015].

Kabbah, President A.A.T. (2000) *Address to the Parliament, 16 June 2000.* Available at: http://www.sierra-leone.org/Speeches/kabbah-061600.html [Accessed 5 August 2015].

Karimu, F. (2001) A green light at the end of a long tunnel, *Young Men's Christian Association Newsletter.* Sierra Leone.

Keen, D. (2005) *The best of enemies: Conflict and collusion in Sierra Leone.* Oxford: James Currey Ltd.

Kelsall, T. (2004) *Truth, lies and ritual: Preliminary reflections on the TRC in Sierra Leone.* Paper presented at the Debating Africa conference, London.

Krech, R. (2003) *The reintegration of former child combatants: A case study of NGO programming in Sierra Leone.* Toronto: University of Toronto.

Liechty, J. (1998) History and reconciliation: Frank Wright, Whitley Stokes, and the vortex of antagonism. In A. Falconer, J. Liechty (Eds.), *Reconciling memories* (2nd ed., pp. 149–176). Dublin: The Columba Press.

Limbs of Hope (2001) *Technical report on the impact of the amputee care centre.* Freetown, Sierra Leone: World Hope International.

Lorey, B., Beezley, W. (2002) *Genocide, collective violence, and popular memory: The politics of remembrance in the twentieth century.* Wilmington, DE: Scholarly Resources Inc.

Montville, J. V. (1993) The healing function in political conflict resolution. In D. J. Sandole, H. van der Merwe (Eds.), *Conflict resolution theory and practice: Integration and application* (pp. 112–127). Manchester: Manchester University Press.

Mundy, L. (2005) The role of traditional ritual in peacebuilding: With examples from Sierra Leone and Israel-Palestine. Unpublished Master of Arts in Conflict Resolution, University of Bradford, United Kingdom.

Murphy, J. G., Hampton, J. (1988) *Forgiveness and mercy.* Cambridge: Cambridge University Press.

Rieber, C. (1977) Traditional Christianity as an African religion. In N. S. Booth (Ed.), *African religions: A symposium* (pp. 255–274). New York: NOK Publishers.

Salia, S. K. (Ed.) (2000) *Friends again*. Freetown: The Council of Churches in Sierra Leone.

Shaw, R. (2004a) *The heart of the matter: Reconciling ex-combatants in Sierra Leone's TRC*. Paper presented at the Debating Africa conference, London.

Shaw, R. (2004b) *Forgive and forget: Rethinking memory in Sierra Leone's Truth and Reconciliation Commission*. Washington, DC: United States Institute for Peace.

Shriver, D. (1995) *An ethic for enemies: Forgiveness in politics*. Oxford: Oxford University Press.

Shriver, D. (2003) Where and when in political life is justice served by forgiveness? In N. Biggar (Ed.), *Burying the past: Making peace and doing justice after civil conflict* (2nd ed., pp. 25–44). Washington, DC: Georgetown University Press.

TRC (Truth and Reconciliation Commission) (2004) *Witness to the truth: Report of Sierra Leone Truth and Reconciliation Commission*. Freetown: TRC and Witness.

Turay, T. M. (2000) Civil society and peacebuilding: The role of the Inter-religious Council of Sierra Leone. Available at: www.cr.org.sites/default/files/Accord%2009_10Civil%20 society%20and%20peacebuilding_2000_ENG.pdf [Accessed 20 April 2015].

Van Deusen Hunsinger, D. (2001) Forgiving abusive parents: Psychological and theological considerations. In A. McFadyen, M. Sarot (Eds.), *Forgiveness and truth* (pp. 71–98). Edinburgh: T & T Clark.

Voeten, T. (2000) *How de body?* (R. Vatter-Buck, Trans.). New York: St. Martin's Press.

Volf, M. (1996) *Exclusion and embrace: A theological exploration of identity, otherness and reconciliation*. Nashville: Abingdon Press.

Williamson, J., Cripe, L. (2002) *Assessment of DCOF-supported child demobilization and reintegration activities in Sierra Leone*. Washington, DC: US Agency for International Development.

Willmer, H. (2003) Jesus Christ the forgiven: Christology, atonement and forgiveness. In A. McFadyen, M. Sarot (Eds.), *Forgiveness and truth* (pp. 15–29). Edinburgh: T & T Clark.

Worthington Jr, E. (1998) The pyramid model of forgiveness: Some interdisciplinary speculations about unforgiveness and the promotion of forgiveness. In E. L. Worthington Jr (Ed.), *Dimensions of forgiveness: Psychological research and religious perspectives* (pp. 107–137). Philadelphia: Templeton Foundation Press.

Worthington Jr, E. (2005) *Handbook of forgiveness*. New York: Routledge.

Wright, F. (1998) Northern Ireland and the British-Irish relationship. In A. Falconer, J. Liechty (Eds.), *Reconciling memories* (2nd ed., pp. 248–260). Dublin: The Columba Press.

Wright, N. T. (1996) *Jesus and the victory of God*. London: Society for Promoting Christian Knowledge.

# Chapter 14

# Culture, society and ways of understanding

*When the music changes, so does the dance.*

(African proverb)

Chapter 11 considered the current mental health provision in Sierra Leone and the recent initiatives as part of the global mental health agenda (GMHA). The discussion brought to the foreground the challenging dilemmas inherent in this movement. The preceding chapters have also highlighted, as other authors have (Brown, 2013; Fernando, 2012; Summerfield, 2001), the overarching void in considering the role of culture and context within research, intervention programmes, and the wider GMHA. The biomedical model of mental health dominates and risks 'chaining' alternative ways of understanding and responding.

This chapter will consider how dominant ways of understanding such matters as trauma, mental health problems and forgiveness may both guide and constrain people's responses and choices in post-conflict situations. Developing arguments from previous chapters, and drawing upon the authors' personal reflections, there will be critical discussion of the GMHA, and the appropriateness of its concepts and methods, in an African context. Suggestions will also be provided for the most appropriate responses and research methods to use in such a context.

## Chained stories, power and distress

The research presented in Chapter 8 has highlighted how the dominant discourses in Sierra Leone (because of almighty God, we forgive; bear it, and forget) may have provided both a guide and a chain to the stories people were able to tell about how they coped and managed following civil war. The discussion of this research considered the influence of chained stories upon the trajectory of the narrative and the emotional distress displayed by individuals and communities. The consideration of the impact of political and societal inequality upon distress, what we call mental illness, has been introduced, and will now be further developed by exploring the influence of power in relation to the biomedical model and GMHA. As Mills (2014) highlights, issues of power are central to any discussion of global mental health.

Foucault (1982) talked about illegitimate discourses, how the complex power relationships in every aspect of our social, cultural and political lives can lead us to internalize the norms and values that prevail within the social order. Therefore, some discourses remain 'illegitimate' or silenced. The LUUUTT model within the theory of Coordinated Management of Meaning (CMM; Pearce, 1999) also encompasses this conceptualization. LUUUTT is an acronym for 1) stories **L**ived, 2) **U**nknown stories, 3) **U**ntold Stories, 4) **U**nheard stories, 5) stories **T**old, and 6) story **T**elling. The LUUUTT model considers *stories lived* as the co-constructed patterns of joint actions that we and others perform, whereas *stories told* are the explanatory narratives that people use to make sense of stories lived (Pearce, 1999). In considering the richness of communication, the LUUUTT model also focuses on the *unknown stories* which are not currently possible to tell, in contrast to *untold stories*, which the participants are capable of telling but have chosen not to. *Unheard stories* are those which, although they have been told, have not been heard. CMM suggests that a spiralling process may unfold, where unheard stories become untold stories, and untold stories become, after a while, unknown stories (Pearce, 1999).

What happens to untold and unknown stories; the stories that are chained? In the research described in Chapter 8, an example of an untold and unknown story was conceptualized during the analysis as '*Why, God?*'. This was in comparison to the dominant storyline of '*Because of Almighty God, We Forgive*'. Whilst the less dominant storyline '*Why, God?*' was present in some of the stories, it was not explicitly mentioned in all the narratives. This could be interpreted in one of two ways. Firstly, the absence of 'Why, God?' could be because no one else had asked this question. Alternatively, another viewpoint is that in the context of Sierra Leone, where religion is interlinked with society, explicit questioning of this discourse could lead to further social rejection. It seems in this context that explicitly questioning God is seen to be associated with, or permitted by, 'madness'. As Emily Dickinson (1998) writes,

> Much Madness is divinest Sense –
> To a discerning Eye –
> Much Sense – the starkest Madness –
> 'Tis the Majority
> In this, as all, prevail –
> Assent – and you are sane –
> Demur – you're straightway dangerous –
> And handled with a Chain
>
> (p. 613)

Questioning God may be seen as going against the political drive for peace and reconciliation. Shuman (2005) argues that the conditions that make a story tellable or untellable rely on socially accepted categories and unrecognizable or unacceptable categories. This research supports existing ideas that culture defines what can be known and told. Consequently the untold or the 'chained' narratives remain without an audience and therefore in an un-storied form; they remain in chaos. It is the social context, the inequality in what kind of stories are accepted and unaccepted, which relates to levels of distress that we then call mental illness. This is a stark alternative to ideas within affluent individualist cultures such as the United Kingdom and United States, where distress is conceptualized as primarily relating to a biological impairment. Alternatively, current evidence is demonstrating (Marmot, 2013; Wilkinson & Pickett, 2010) that the social context, inequality, poverty and power are highly relevant factors in the creation of what we call mental health problems. Changes in biology may then come as a consequence, but the efficacy of pharmacological treatments is under question (Speed, Moncrieff & Rapley, 2014).

The questions and critical reviews which surround the dominant ideas currently influencing the mental health systems in high-resource, individualistic cultures are imperative to consider as the GMHA unfolds. There is recognition that sharing some ideas and practices from 'high-resource' countries could be useful, but only if cultural context is placed strictly in the foreground and careful and critical reflection on the applicability of ideas is central. Understanding how issues of power are unfolding within the GMHA is an ethical imperative for all involved.

## The global mental health agenda

The field of global health places a priority on improving health and achieving equity for all people worldwide (Patel & Prince, 2010). The global mental health agenda (GMHA) can therefore be seen as driven to apply these principles to the domain of mental health. Much controversy surrounds the concepts of 'mental health' and 'mental illness', and the models of understanding individual and collective distress. There are significant questions and dilemmas about what ethical and emic[1] mental health systems might look like.

Mental health around the world has now become a central concern for health organizations: 'No health without mental health' (World Health Organization [WHO], 2005). Furthermore, the WHO Comprehensive Mental Health Action Plan was adopted by the WHO World Health Assembly in May 2013. This followed recognition of mental health as an essential component of the global health agenda, including within non-communicable diseases. Fernando (2012) describes how key papers in the *Lancet* series on global mental health (e.g., Prince et al., 2007) attest to the importance of attending to mental health issues when considering overall health. The series culminates in a call to action for scaling up resources for mental health, including improvements in funding, policy and personnel (Lancet Global Mental Health Group, 2007). This resulted in the development of a coalition called the Movement for Global Mental Health (MGMH), which is described as an international coalition of professionals and the public who are committed to improving access to mental health care and promoting the human rights of people affected by mental illness worldwide. This coalition is influential with policy makers, but significant criticism has evolved around it, a key voice being that of China Mills (2014), who describes the movement as a neocolonial project to globalize Western psychiatry.

### The medicalization of difference

The Movement for Global Mental Health can be seen to be advocating for the transfer of mental health systems that have been developed in affluent, individualistic cultures to low-resource cultures that may not hold an individualist frame for understanding experience. The language of 'mental disorder' and diagnostic categories such as schizophrenia is widely used within their publications. This is despite the current concerns about the efficacy of the biomedical model (Smail, 2005; Speed et al., 2014). Indeed, Mills (2014) questions the role that the pharmaceutical industry plays within GMHA, and asks why the MGMH does not engage in transparent discussion about the wider political economy of scaling up. Fernando (2012) points out that the 2007 *Lancet* papers do not consider sufficiently the influence of context and culture upon the development and maintenance of distress. Isakson and Jurkovic (2013) also make this point in the research around healing after torture. They highlight that the experience and sociocultural context of torture and its treatment have received little attention in the biopsychosocial model of Western, high-resource mental health for survivors of torture. Results from their research showed that stories of moving on and healing were not centred on individual symptom reduction but on social, interpersonal, spiritual, ethical and sociopolitical healing. Participants described being able to move on and function more adaptively despite continuing psychological distress which would fit the categories of PTSD, anxiety and depression.

### Is 'severe mental health problems' a useful and ethical label?

Mills (2014) points out that the language commonly used in this field, such as 'disorder' and 'severe mental health problems', may not be a useful or valid way of describing individuals' and communities' experiences of distress. Fernando (2012) also made this point, stating that the term 'mental health', in the way that it is currently used, reflects a bias towards intrapsychic, individual, and dysfunctional processes. In fact there is evidence to show that explanations of distress as being biochemical, and within people's brains, while reducing blame, actually increase stigma, desire for social distance and punitive treatment from the public (Mills, 2014).

The current GMHA discourse is typically produced by psychiatrists in countries high in economic resources, about people in countries low in resources. An alternative definition of global mental health has been proposed by Fernando (2012) as the mental health and mental ill health of people across the globe, experienced and expressed in culturally distinct ways.

The criticism of the GMH movement is not solely centred on the 'scaling up' of medication. A number of authors have highlighted the view that, if unquestioned, the dominant therapeutic approaches in the United Kingdom, and the lack of consideration of the role of culture, could be experienced as racist because they privilege Western concepts of the self and mental health (Fernando, 2012). In the special issue of the Clinical Psychology Forum *Clinical Psychology around the World*, Latchford and Melluish (2010) highlighted a concern that the internationalizing of clinical psychology may lead to the inappropriate export of Western theories and models and the potential marginalization of indigenous knowledge. A number of other authors have critically considered the challenges that can arise when transferring Western models of mental health to low economic resource countries (e.g., White, 2013).

The question, therefore, is centred on whether there might be more useful ways of understanding and intervening (for example, taking seriously conditions of poverty and social inequality). David Smail (2005) coined the phrase that what people need is 'outsight' of the impact of the world around them rather than 'insight'. An alternative approach to GMH would be to bring to the foreground the politicized understandings of distress as linked to, for example, socioeconomic inequalities, and not frameworks that see this as 'illness' within people's brains (Mills, 2014).

The position of psychiatric colonization that individuals and organizations from affluent individualized cultures may find themselves in is challenging and likely a result of benign intention. Through drawing on one of the author's (Rachel's) personal reflection from completing research and providing training within Sierra Leone, consideration will now be directed to how this dynamic may be created.

## 'The desire to help'

'The desire to help' (Brown, 2014) is an externalized phrase developed to reflect the dynamic that researchers and clinicians from affluent individualized countries may experience within their relationship to the global mental health movement. The narrative practice of externalizing views experience and phenomena as socially constructed, as products of culture and history, rather than as within individuals.

During one of the author's (Rachel's) experience within Sierra Leone as a researcher and trainer, she reflected upon her feeling of an uncomfortable and confusing dynamic within the relationships she encountered. She noticed that she was often invited into adopting a powerful position; into the expectation that she could help, that she had the knowledge, resources or money to solve a problem. However, Rachel felt uncomfortable with the idea that Western psychological knowledge was necessarily superior to the resources and understanding held within the communities of people requesting help. She did not want to be seen as a saviour; yet it also seemed unhelpful not to accept this responsibility. Through privilege Rachel felt powerful but nevertheless powerless. The interpersonal inequality between 'helper' and 'requester of help' is important. Miller and McClelland (2006) state that social inequalities are structural differences or hierarchies of power that limit and constrain some people and privilege and empower others. As McIntosh (1990) highlights, racism can be found in the invisible systems that confer dominance. From this perspective the importation of Western models of mental health may be viewed as psychological colonization.

A question which remained in Rachel's mind was:

> What commitments do we wish to make in order to ensure that we respond to our 'desire to help' in an ethical way?

A 'desire to help' may pull us into certain positions, for example the position of 'expert' or 'saviour'. However, as individuals and as a collective we have a choice about how to respond to this temptation. As a number of authors have asserted (e.g., Summerfield, 2001), if we try to provide psychological support and consultation from a position of evolutionism, from the standpoint that our Western knowledge is superior, then we risk disabling the communities we are trying to help. Interestingly, the challenge that Rachel experienced in Sierra Leone was that when she tried to take a different position, for example the position of facilitator or enabler, she felt that this seemed to create uncertainty for the person seeking help. One way of understanding this dynamic may be through the concept of reciprocal roles. In this conceptualization, Ryle and Kerr (2003) described how our early learning about the social world is stored in the form of internalized templates. Within these templates there is a role for the self and a role for the other; for example, the reciprocal role between 'expert' and 'ignorant', or 'saviour' and 'in need of saving'. Ryle and Kerr (2003) also suggest that when an individual adopts one pole in the relationship, the other person can be forced to adopt the congruent pole. Therefore, if those wanting to help accept the position of 'expert' or 'saviour', do we give those we try to help any option of being anything other than 'ignorant' and 'in need of saving'?

## What kind of 'help' would fit an African context?

> Have you come to solve a problem, or are you there to enable others to solve it?
> (Baum and Lynggaard, 2006, p. 162)

The risks, dilemmas and interpersonal dynamics involved in positioning certain models or ways of understanding as 'right' have been highlighted and considered in context. The void in appreciating the role of culture in understanding expressions of distress is key; if we give power to one model of understanding distress (e.g., the biomedical model) above alternative conceptions (e.g., traditional beliefs), the different ways of understanding individual and collective narratives may become constrained and effectively 'chained' in a similar way to how patients at the Sierra Leone Psychiatric Hospital and the City of Rest have historically been chained to their beds. This is an issue of human rights, and the globalization of a medical model of mental health and psychiatric medication is also an issue of human rights, albeit a more invisible one. Instead of furthering well-being, the result of 'scaling up' a biomedical model of mental health in Sierra Leone and beyond may be that over time the distress of such nations will be exacerbated rather than alleviated. Without paying some attention to emic formulations of psychological distress, the scaling up of programs and resources called for by GMH researchers (Lancet Global Mental Health Group, 2007) may only result in more studies that perpetuate the same diagnostic biases and categorical fallacies (Fernando, 2012)

There is a risk that through adopting a critical perspective on the current dominant models inherent within the GMHA, individuals, communities and organizing systems may feel despondent about how best to respond within low economic resource countries. However, researchers and practitioners can and do take positions such as 'facilitator' and 'collaborator'. Most researchers in GMH would agree that community distress is greater than the sum of the distress of its individual members, particularly in collectivistic cultures. For example, Somasundaram (2010) uses the term 'collective trauma'. Mills (2014) begins to outline what an alternative to scaling up models of mental health care that are dominated by psychiatry might look like. She discusses a project of decolonization, revealing and dismantling forms of colonial power – including those that operate through psychiatry – using local and indigenous tools as well as new and creative alliances between diverse groups.

## Culturally anchored responses

The findings from the research discussed in Chapter 8 (Brown, 2014) highlight the importance of the relationship *between* dominant and counter narratives in the maintenance of distress. The historical cultural focus on interdependent understandings of the 'self' and the struggle to make sense of the change in social interactions during and following the civil war were clear. As Bracken, Giller and Summerfield (1995) discuss, war and organized violence often damage traditional ways of life. This damage can mean that the events of the war are even more traumatic for individuals who are left without a meaningful framework in which to structure their suffering. These are often the individuals who find themselves in mental health institutions. Responses to distress need to be culturally anchored and informed by an understanding of what are the available dominant discourses (social, cultural, historical, political) which may be influencing how individuals and communities are able to makes sense out of events that happen to them.

A recommendation from the research discussed in Chapter 8 was that health initiatives should focus on the social reintegration of people in distress back into the community. The focus should be on enabling communities by facilitating alternative understandings of distress rather than 'treating' people in mental health institutions and perpetuating social isolation. This is based on the idea that in a context which historically advocates a 'We Bear It' narrative, social isolation is likely to maintain suffering. The research described in Chapter 7 indicated that untold, unknown and unheard stories play a perpetuating role in the cycle of 'chaos' of expressed distress. The owners of such stories often become labelled as 'mentally unwell', which then often results in social exclusion and expulsion from one's community. A vicious cycle is created between dominant narratives, suppression, distress and exclusion. Consequently, it is relevant to work with individuals' and communities' personal meaning-making processes. This would involve hearing the expression of the less accepted stories, alongside the more socially focused interventions. This does not necessarily mean that 'talking therapies' are the most appropriate way for less accepted stories to be expressed, since there are many creative and culturally congruent ways of expression which may fit African contexts, such as dance, ceremony, story telling and companionable silence.

In Sierra Leone there has been a drive for the reintegration of child soldiers. There may be lessons that could be learnt from these processes to support people experiencing other less culturally acceptable forms of distress. This will be particularly relevant in the aftermath of Ebola. The church and religious leaders have the power to influence social discourse around the conceptualization of distress. The research discussed within this book leads to the recommendation that any attempts to help should be in consultation with the heads of communities and religious leaders in order to develop a space where dialogue about alternative ideas regarding expression of distress can take place. As Mbiti (1975) states, African religion is to be found in all aspects of life; African psychology, therefore, has to embrace African religion. This idea is supported by Fernando (2012), who describes how religious beliefs are intimately associated with psychosocial functioning and mental health in collectivistic cultures, and culturally informed discussions on such issues need to be included in a GMHA if it is to be authentically 'global' in outlook. Isakson and Jurkovic (2013) also outline recommendations for culturally congruent methods of responding following experiences of torture, highlighting the importance of 1) reconstructing cultural institutions, formal and informal social networks, and sources of support; 2) communitywide rebuilding of adaptive systems of health (safety and security, attachment, justice, existential meaning, and identity/role); 3) using indigenous healers and rituals that mobilize culturally based resiliency and coping strategies related to mourning and purification; and 4) drawing on religious and spiritual beliefs and practices to make meaning of and to ameliorate the survivor's suffering.

Finally, the relationship between poverty, inequality and what we refer to as mental distress is widely discussed through this book. In line with this understanding, a culturally congruent response to supporting the mental health of low-resource countries may be to work towards alleviating the conditions of poverty and inequality first and foremost.

## What would culturally anchored research look like?

Despite the highlighted importance of culture, it is clear that even large-scale global surveys often fail to consider cultural beliefs in their design of studies and their publications. An example is the World Mental Health Survey Initiative. In this multisite, multicountry study, researchers intentionally planned to address cultural variations in assessment and diagnosis, via face-to-face structured diagnostic interviews. Of the more than 500 subsequent publications, however, fewer than 25 explicitly examine the cross-cultural validity of the assessment interview and format used in the study (Fernando, 2012). As discussed in Chapter 10, if research programmes set research questions and methodology from an etic[2] framework, then research findings will reflect an etic understanding of experience. Alternatively, what is required is a culturally anchored and congruent research agenda for global mental health. In support, Monteiro and Balogun (2014) discuss how questions are now being raised regarding whether assumptions underlying the paradigms, approaches and methodology used in large-scale quantitative and population research are appropriate for all settings, groups and research inquiries. The question becomes, are the methods used in broad survey or epidemiological analysis adequate to address the ways that culture impacts research procedures and interpretation of results? Monteiro and Balogun (2014) go on to indicate how some mental health researchers have highlighted the importance of considering and attending to culture at every stage of research, from conceptualization and formulation of research questions to implementation of methods and procedures, and interpretation of findings.

Community participatory research and qualitative research are highlighted by Monteiro and Balogun (2014) as best practice. Community participatory research is a methodology where researchers work in partnership with communities in a manner that leads to action for change. It stems from a perspective that the most accurate and useful information is acquired when there is a collaborative relationship with and strong participation from the community. There is also the assumption that embedded in the research design is the goal of providing some outcome benefit to the community. Factors such as obtaining buy-in from marginalized communities, encouraging participation in research that is relevant to the target community, developing culturally congruent research questions and procedures, and liaising with government and official ministerial and other community stakeholders are key to developing culturally congruent methodology (Monteiro & Balogun, 2014). A reflective process is directly linked to action, influenced by an understanding of history, culture and local context, which is embedded in social relationships (Baum & Lynggaard, 2006). Walker, Johnson and Cunningham (2012) highlight that community participatory research might offer a new mode of transformative practice in relation to mental health on the global stage.

Fernando (2012) reflects that it is probably not a coincidence that attention to culture is lacking in the prevailing discourses on GMH when the majority of professionals currently engaged in developing the GMHA are raised and/or trained in high-resource, individualized cultures. Unfortunately, only about 10 per cent of published papers in mental health are authored by researchers not living and working in such cultures. Researchers invested in cultural conceptualizations of mental health tend to favor qualitative studies, but the scientific readership may not consider these to be as valuable as quantitative studies (Kirmayer, 2006).

## Conclusion

This chapter has provided an overview of the GMHA and a critical discussion on the role of power in the creation of distress. This has involved reflecting on the relational dynamics between helper and those requesting help. The question 'What kind of help would fit an African context?' has been explored, and ideas for culturally anchored research responses have been outlined. There are unfortunately no certainties or 'truths' to be concluded at the end of this discussion but for the suggestion that the dilemmas outlined need to be actively engaged with in order to ensure both ethical responses for those wishing to 'help' and the fundamental protection of human rights as those with power attempt to assist those with less power. The lessons learnt from the research and discussion throughout this book will now be explored in further depth in Chapter 15.

## Notes

1  An emic approach investigates how local people perceive and experience the world, their rules for behaviour, what has meaning for them, and how they imagine and explain things.
2  From the perspective of a culture other than the one studied.

## References

Baum, S., Lynggaard, H. (Eds.) (2006) *Intellectual disabilities: A systemic approach.* London: Karnac.

Bracken, P. J., Giller, J. E., Summerfield, D. (1995) Psychological responses to war and atrocity: the limitations of current concepts. *Social Science & Medicine,* 40(8): 1073–1082.

Brown, R. (2013) *'I fall down, I get up': Stories of survival and resistance following civil war in Sierra Leone.* Unpublished doctoral thesis, University of Hertfordshire, United Kingdom.

Brown, R. (2014) The desire to help in low economic countries. *Clinical Psychology Forum,* 258: 19–22.

Dickinson, E. (1998) *The Poems of Emily Dickinson* (Vol. 1) (R. W. Franklin, Ed.). Cambridge, MA: Belknap Press.

Fernando, G. A. (2012) The roads less traveled: Mapping some pathways on the global mental health research roadmap. *Transcultural Psychiatry,* 49: 396–417.

Foucault, M. (1982) The subject and power. *Critical Inquiry,* 8(4): 777–795.

Isakson, B. L., Jurkovic, G. J. (2013) Healing after torture the role of moving on. *Qualitative Health Research,* 23(6): 749–761.

Kirmayer, L. J. (2006). Beyond the 'new cross-cultural psychiatry': Cultural biology, discursive psychology and the ironies of globalization. *Transcultural Psychiatry,* 43(1): 126–144.

Lancet Global Mental Health Group (2007) Scale up services for mental disorders: A call for action. *The Lancet,* 370(9594): 1241–1252.

Latchford, G., Melluish, S. (2010) Clinical psychology around the world: An introduction to the special issue. *Clinical Psychology Forum,* 215: 9–11.

Marmot, M. (2013) Fair society, healthy lives. In N. Eyal, S. A. Hurst, O. F. Norheim, D. Wikler (Eds.), *Inequalities in health: Concepts, measures, and ethics* (pp. 282–299). Oxford: Oxford University Press.

Mbiti, J. S. (1975) *Concepts of God in Africa.* London: S.P.C.K.

McIntosh, P. (1990) White privilege: Unpacking the invisible knapsack. *Independent School,* 49(2), 31–36.

Miller, J., McClelland, L. (2006) Social inequalities formulation: Mad, bad and dangerous to know. In L. Johnstone, R. Dallos (Eds.), *Formulation in psychology and psychotherapy: Making sense of people's problems* (pp. 126–154). London: Routledge.

Mills, C. (2014) *Decolonizing global mental health: The psychiatrization of the majority world.* London and New York: Routledge.

Monteiro, N. M., Balogun, S. K. (2014) Culturally congruent mental health research in Africa: Field notes from Ethiopia and Senegal. *African Journal of Psychiatry,* 17: 520–524.

Patel, V., Prince, M. (2010) Global mental health: A new global health field comes of age. *JAMA,* 303(19): 1976–1977.

Pearce, W. B. (1999) *The coordinated management of meaning.* A Pearce Associates seminar. Available at: http://www.pearceassociates.com/essays/cmm_seminar.pdf [Accessed 15 May 2013].

Prince, M., Patel, V., Saxena, S., Maj, M., Maselko, J., Phillips, M. R., Rahman, A. (2007) No health without mental health. *The Lancet,* 370(9590): 859–877.

Ryle, A., Kerr, I. B. (2003) *Introducing cognitive analytic therapy: Principles and practice.* Chichester: Wiley.

Shuman, A. (2005) *Other people's stories: Entitlement claims and the critique of empathy.* Urbana: University of Illinois Press.

Smail, D. J. (2005) *Power, interest and psychology: Elements of a social materialist understanding of distress.* London: PCCS Books.

Somasundaram, D. (2010) Suicide bombers of Sri Lanka. *Asian Journal of Social Science,* 38(3): 416–441.

Speed, E., Moncrieff, J., Rapley, M. (Eds.) (2014) *De-medicalizing misery II: Society, politics and the mental health industry.* West Sussex: Palgrave Macmillan.

Summerfield, D. (2001) The intervention of post-traumatic stress disorder and the social usefulness of a psychiatric category. *British Medical Journal,* 322: 95–98.

Walker, C., Johnson, K., Cunningham, L. (Eds.) (2012) *Community psychology and the socio-economics of mental distress: International perspectives.* New York: Palgrave Macmillan.

White, R. (2013) The globalisation of mental illness. *The Psychologist,* 26(3): 183–185.

WHO (2005) *No health without mental health.* Available at: https://www.gov.uk/government/uploads/system/uploads/attachment_data/file/213761/dh_124058.pdf [Accessed 3 February 2015].

Wilkinson, R., Pickett, K. (2010) *Spirit level* (2nd ed.). London: Allen Lane.

# Chapter 15

# Lessons learnt

*The house owner knows where his house leaks.*
Koranko proverb (Hinzen, James, Sorie & Tamu, 1987, p. 198)

We shall now consider what conclusions and lessons we can draw from our research and the stories that we have been told in relation not just to the situation in Sierra Leone but to that in other countries faced with, or recovering from, armed conflict. We shall discuss implications for appropriate research methods; conceptions of trauma and responses to this; the provision of services for people in psychological distress; the understanding of violence; the healing of communities following conflict; and more generally the provision of aid.

## Research methods

The research that we have presented has used a range of methods, but all consistent with a constructivist or social constructionist epistemological position, namely that individuals and societies construct their views of themselves and their worlds, with constructions being influenced and constrained by the dominant discourses within different societies. As indicated in the previous chapter, the research focus has been on elucidating these constructions in an 'emic' manner rather than viewing the individuals and societies concerned from the perspective of some external, 'etic' framework. The principal methods adopted have been derived from personal construct theory or narrative inquiry, and our research has demonstrated their utility in cultural settings different from that of the researchers – particularly in those, such as Sierra Leone, with a rich oral tradition – and their capacity to help war survivors, both adults and children, tell their stories.

Narrative methods were also used by Bolten (2012) in her study of survivors of the civil war in Sierra Leone, in which she explained the genesis of the war and the behaviours of those involved in it in terms of the polarity of 'love', in the sense of the material loyalty that is highly valued in Sierra Leone, and 'eating', in which resources are greedily hoarded rather than shared. For example, as Bolten describes, the RUF fostered 'love' and loyalty in the alternative 'family' that they provided for their recruits, as well as a view that 'di rotin sistem' against which they fought was characterized by 'eating'. Bolten (2012) addresses the criticism of narrative approaches that the stories told by research participants may not be factual, particularly in a country such as Sierra Leone in which 'A story only becomes a *good* story if you add something to it' (p. 245). She considers that, although all of her narrators were concerned to emphasize their righteousness and capacity for 'love', their stories were nevertheless 'true' in reflecting their reconstructions of their worlds. This is what Kelly (1955) would describe as a 'credulous attitude', in which people's stories are taken at face value. As in previous research on perpetrators of extreme violence, including homicide, this does not necessarily involve agreeing with the narrator's story, but merely taking it seriously and thereby trying to see the world through the other person's eyes.

While issues concerning the veracity of accounts are also raised by the narrative approaches used in some of our studies, these have in some cases been complemented by the use of personal construct methods, such as repertory grid technique, that may access aspects of construing at a lower level of awareness (Winter, 1992) and therefore be less subject to questions about the credibility of their results, than story-telling methods. However, as indicated, for example, in Chapter 8, the latter methods are also able to reveal different levels of storying: from dominant discourses to personal stories that may be 'chained' by these, or that are 'unknown', 'untold', or 'unheard'. We would, in any case, contend that these methods are much more likely to provide a rich and authentic account of a person's situation than a method such as a questionnaire with items that may be of little personal relevance to research participants. Similarly, the relevance to the individual respondent of personal construct methods is assured by the flexibility of these methods, which can be adapted to particular research questions and participants, and in which the constructs explored are those of the individuals concerned, whatever their cultural setting, rather than constructs imposed by the researcher.[1]

## Responses to conflict and trauma

The stories that we have been told have indicated that in Sierra Leone, just as in many other countries plagued by conflict,[2] trauma is part of life. In such countries, as we have discussed in Chapter 10, what would constitute a traumatic event to many Western people may be no more than an everyday occurrence, albeit still an unpleasant and distressing one. Such specific events during the civil war may have been less difficult to deal with in Sierra Leone than the total breakdown of law and order, vividly described in the stories recounted in Part 2 of this book, caused by the overthrow of family and cultural structures, and the blurring of conventional boundaries, or in some cases reversals of power differentials, between, for example, adults and children, government soldiers and rebels, army commanders and their troops, community leaders and common people, and victims and perpetrators of violence. There was also breakdown of moral structures, such as by child soldiers being rewarded for carrying out actions that would previously have been proscribed and deplored, or punished for actions for which previously they might have been praised. In personal construct terms, the situation was one that would have involved a comprehensive invalidation of core constructs and dislodgement of individuals from their core roles, and been experienced in terms of threat, anxiety and guilt, or indeed the sheer confusion and terror that it was intended to instil. Arguably, this is the legacy of the war with which it has been hardest for Sierra Leoneans to come to terms, as in accounts by some of our participants of difficulties in the rebuilding of family bonds following the war (although equally there were many stories of, for example, former child soldiers being reintegrated into their families, while others, as described in Chapter 4, regarded the breakdown of the family as preceding, and a causal factor in, the war). As indicated in Chapter 9, that a 'medical model' focus on past traumatic events may be too simplistic in paying insufficient attention to the difficulties of daily living is also highlighted by the situation of refugees who are having to negotiate possibly no less traumatic current, post-migration issues such as asylum processes.

A further recurrent message from our studies is the questioning of the appropriateness of privileging Western notions of post-traumatic stress, post-traumatic growth and resilience, or indeed other Western psychiatric diagnostic constructs, in describing the varied responses to adversity of people in Africa or other non-Western cultures. As we have described in Chapters 2, 3, and 10, such constructs tend to be based on an intrapsychic view of the self, and can lead to insufficient attention being paid to the individual's social, cultural, historical and political context. The appropriateness of the medicalization of ever more aspects of human experience by the use of these diagnostic constructs[3] even in countries in the Western setting in which they originated can, of course, also be questioned, but this is beyond the scope of the present book.

## Mental health service provision

Our research, as described in Chapters 7 and 11, has highlighted the minimal resources available for people in psychological distress in Sierra Leone, as in many economically deprived countries, sometimes leading to such people being treated in ways which from a Western perspective might be considered inhumane. However, as indicated in the previous section, it has also cautioned against 'psychiatric colonization', the too ready use of Western models of diagnosis and treatment of 'mental health problems', in a setting such as Sierra Leone.

This can best be illustrated by again considering responses to 'trauma'. In the Western context, there has been a shift from the promotion of rapid intervention following trauma, using approaches such as critical stress debriefing, to a realization that such interventions may in fact be counterproductive in that they may reduce the rate of post-trauma recovery, perhaps by lessening the extent to which people make use of their natural social resources in coming to terms with traumatic events. Indeed, critical stress debriefing has moved from being championed to being included in a list of potentially 'harmful' therapies (Lilienfeld, 2007). Nevertheless, there is still a tendency following situations of armed conflict, terrorism, or natural disaster to mobilize therapeutic and training packages provided by a veritable army of Western experts in post-traumatic stress disorder (Watters, 2010).

As we have seen in Chapter 2, positive trajectories following adversity are not uncommon, with resilience being the norm, and a more helpful approach than automatically reaching for the Western PTSD treatment manual may be to facilitate the use of the local resources and practices that promote such trajectories and to learn from local examples of resilience. More generally, what is required in Sierra Leone, as in many other countries, is greater recognition, not only by the general public but also by some staff members working with such individuals, of the humanity of people in psychological distress. Labelling such people as mentally ill and medicating them may not serve this purpose if it only reinforces the distinction between them and us and makes it less likely that attempts are made to understand, and take seriously, their view of the world and the role of socioeconomic factors in their distress.

## Understanding violence

In this book we have argued that it is not only the person in psychological distress who needs to be understood but also (in the interest of working towards the prevention of further violence) the person who commits acts of extreme violence. In Chapter 4, we have highlighted some of the social, political and historical factors underlying the civil war in Sierra Leone and the atrocities that occurred during this war, and at an individual level, in Chapters 5 and 12, we have also tried to glimpse the world through the eyes of the person who commits such atrocities, whether this be a child soldier or someone who makes a freer choice to inflict suffering on others. To do so is not an entirely comfortable process as it involves acknowledging that the horrific acts that were committed in Sierra Leone are not, as they are sometimes portrayed, merely an expression of African barbarism and savagery but that they are not dissimilar to those perpetrated in other armed conflicts, including by people from the more 'developed' world. Understanding the perspective of the person who commits violence, just like understanding that of the person who might be labelled mentally ill, can also be threatening as it implies that their psychological processes are essentially no different to our own. This certainly does not mean that we have to condone the perspectives of people who commit violence, nor does it mean that we would ever behave in the same way, but we might nevertheless have to ask ourselves how we would have responded if placed in the same situation as a child soldier in Sierra Leone.

## Social recovery

Understanding of the perspective of the other is central to approaches to recovery and reconciliation following wrongdoing such as restorative justice (Tschudi, 2016). In Sierra Leone, as in some other countries following conflict, the approach taken to rebuilding of the community after the civil war has tended to be one of prescribed forgiveness (sometimes after prescribed requests for forgiveness by perpetrators of violence), as discussed in Chapter 13. Although, as we have seen in the stories presented in Part 2, there have certainly been several examples of individuals expressing the dominant discourse that, in the interests of peace in their country, they will forgive even those who have caused them intense suffering, at another level some seemed to tell a somewhat different story. Indeed, the position taken by most of our research participants seemed to be that they would forgive but would never forget – and, indeed, how could one easily forget the loss of one's limb, one's loved ones, one's livelihood, one's self-respect, and one's dreams?

While accepting that forgiveness is central to community healing and reintegration following conflict, our view is that it can neither be forced nor rushed. In the examples that we have provided, forgiveness has most effectively been promoted by approaches that have drawn upon traditional practices such as rituals, ceremonies and story telling.

## Aid

That aid, either in terms of financial and material resources or personnel and training, should be provided to a country, like Sierra Leone, that is faced with the massive hardship of recovering from a conflict or natural catastrophe may often seem self-evident. However, as we have seen in Chapters 4, 11 and 14, the nature and extent of such aid requires careful consideration. The aid industry is big business, and one which arguably causes both donors and recipients to have a vested interest in at some level colluding in the maintenance of conflicts. In Sierra Leone, as described by Keen (2005), the government and other 'big men' clearly benefited greatly from the provision of aid, and the siphoning of this away from those for whom it was (at least ostensibly) intended allowed the maintenance of existing systems of patronage, fuelled resentment amongst those who failed to benefit from it, and ultimately perpetuated the war. Following the war, further resentment ensued from a perception that aid was channelled towards the reintegration into society of perpetrators of violence with relatively little attention to the needs of the victims of that violence.

As Maathai (2009) has described, aid programmes may also, by essentially treating symptoms rather than helping countries to develop longer-term solutions to their problems, promote dependence rather than empowerment. This may be particularly so in Africa, the colonial history of which has, in Maathai's view, left Africans with a 'cultural inferiority complex', which has only been exacerbated by its dependence on aid from its former colonial powers and by the images of suffering, poverty and helplessness that are commonly portrayed in the rest of the world by the media and in fund-raising campaigns. There is therefore a constant fostering of passivity, and of the belief, as we have seen in previous chapters, that people 'will ultimately be saved by an outside force rather than by the sum of their actions' (Maathai, 2009, p. 40). The aid industry may thus be viewed as a form of neocolonialism since, to quote Maathai (2009, p. 108) again, 'In the past, people entered Africa by force. These days, they come with similarly lethal packages, but they are camouflaged attractively to persuade Africa's leaders and peoples to cooperate', and there is 'a continuation of the dynamic whereby the industrialized world provides Africa with assistance and removes its natural capital on the other' (p. 279). There is therefore still a 'systematic theft of Africa's wealth' (Burgis, 2015), albeit more subtle, but perhaps consequently more dangerous, than in the colonial era. In this process, African heads of state are increasingly turning to new 'friends' in countries, such as China, that were not their former colonial powers. Roads and buildings are duly and rapidly constructed, education and training programmes are provided, but at the same time there is environmental destruction and pollution, and Africa's natural resources are stripped even further, as are its human assets, the newly trained professionals often emigrating to work in the countries that provided the resources for their training. When one of us (David) taught community health officers in Sierra Leone, the most eagerly anticipated and best-attended session was always the one at which the students were presented with certificates of attendance, seen by many as possible passports to working overseas. David was also saddened on one of his visits to Freetown to find that his favourite little makeshift bars and restaurants where one could watch the sun set on Lumley Beach had been closed down, ostensibly in the interests of beautifying the beach but more likely to attempt to force foreign visitors to frequent and spend their money in the concrete monstrosities that had been built by Sierra Leone's new 'friends' on the other side of the street. The foundations of many such new constructions are shaky in every sense, and Africa's leaders may be well advised to heed some of their continent's traditional wisdom, for example:

> *There are different kinds of friendship: A cowdung friendship has cement on the surface, while the bottom holds a pool of water.*
>
> Mende proverb (Hinzen et al., 1987, p. 149)

A further problem with the provision of technical aid and training, which two of us experienced when attempting to provide input to Sierra Leone Psychiatric Hospital, concerns the sustainability of any changes introduced after the aid providers or trainers have left. This problem arises partly from the culture of dependency, but also from local people not being actively involved in the development of the solutions to their own problems. For example, as described in Chapter 11, although provision of training by Western delegations may lead to some short-term gains in terms of instituting new practices, it is unlikely that these will be sustained unless local workers have a sense of ownership of, and investment in, these practices. Similarly, while offers of equipment will rarely be refused, perhaps partly because the recipients do not wish to cause offence, whether the equipment will continue to be used after the donors leave is another matter. Offers of aid in the form of new equipment or training programmes may therefore at an overt level be effusively welcomed, but more covertly there may be rejection of the aid – perhaps partly because of it being viewed as another example of cultural imperialism – in that there is a return to old practices as soon as the donors are no longer present. One of us (David) is aware of a situation in which a visiting medic was so appalled by the outdated and poorly functioning equipment in a Sierra Leone hospital that she arranged at her own considerable expense for a new machine to be transported to Sierra Leone from her own country. On its arrival, she was then surprised to receive a bill for customs duty and for the transportation of the equipment from the port of arrival to the hospital. She nevertheless paid the bill, but some considerable time later the equipment has still not been, and is probably never likely to be, removed from its packaging.

The most recent influx of aid workers to Sierra Leone has been in response to the Ebola crisis. This has involved many brave health professionals, who have at times put their own safety at risk in working with victims of the disease. While such efforts are to be applauded, their implementation has also at times highlighted some of the dangers of not taking sufficient heed of local beliefs and practices. For example, the sudden arrival of workers in protective 'space suits' in remote villages to take away Ebola sufferers often only fed into beliefs concerning evil spirits, or that Ebola was a Western or government[4] plot to gain money. Such beliefs are similar to those that had previously been reported in Sierra Leone and elsewhere in Africa concerning HIV infection and AIDS. Whether or not Ebola aid provision brought any financial benefits, it was certainly as much focused on containing the spread of the disease, including to the Western world, as on helping those affected by it in Sierra Leone and other African countries.

We would emphasize that it is certainly not our intention to minimize the immense suffering that has been endured by the people of Sierra Leone or of other countries that have endured warfare, or the need for this suffering to be ameliorated. Nor do we question that the vast majority of those who provide aid are entirely well meaning. We merely urge awareness and minimization of the possible neocolonial aspects of this situation. As discussed in Chapter 14, we have not been without our own dilemmas when carrying out the work reported in this book, for example in relation to our 'desire to help' in Sierra Leone. We are also, of course, not immune to the criticism that we have exploited Sierra Leonean people by using their stories to further our careers or promote our favoured models. We are acutely aware that we all come from privileged Western backgrounds. However, as well as our research participants effectively acting as co-researchers, we have consulted widely with people from Sierra Leone, several of whom we have acknowledged in the Preface, during our research. We can do no more than try to be aware of the dangers of ethnocentrically imposing our views and to take care not to distort the stories that we have been told. We leave it to the reader to judge how successful we have been in this.

## Conclusions

A common message from the studies reported in this book is that, in recovering from a situation of armed conflict, either at an individual or at a societal level, the approaches that are most likely to succeed are those that are locally driven, drawing upon the resources of local people and their indigenous practices and cultural and religious beliefs. This does not mean that there is no room for learning from Western ideas and techniques, but care should be taken to integrate these with traditional beliefs and to ensure that local people are fully involved in, and 'signed up to', their implementation. There should also be mindfulness of the power held by the Western professional who tries to introduce particular ideas, and of whether local people have the power to reject or disagree with these ideas. In other words, there should be no imposition of a dominant Western discourse and concomitant silencing of local discourses, but instead, as Maathai (2009) has urged, Africans should help themselves by 'reclaiming their culture' rather than depending upon Western practices and experts. Equally, Western professionals should be aware that they may again and again be invited into the position of expert, and that it is their ethical duty to endeavour to resist this position as this is the only way to afford the 'other' the opportunity to share their knowledge and skills. As a Kenyan man passionately proclaimed at a conference that one of us (Stephanie) attended some years ago, 'We do not need your resources or your expertise. We have all that within us. What we need is your support.'

It is for such reasons that, while the delegation with which two of us have been involved in providing training in Sierra Leone has perhaps contributed to reducing the practice of chaining in the psychiatric hospital, the group's attention has now turned towards encouraging trained Sierra Leonean mental health workers in the United Kingdom to return to their country and help to develop its services. The potential of native Sierra Leoneans, even without training, to promote individual and community recovery is indicated by the fact that two of the most effective interventions described by our participants, the amputee football team and the Community Theatre Agency, were initiatives developed by local people. These interventions unknowingly exemplified some of the principles of therapeutic techniques used in the Western world,[5] but they crucially paid due attention to the vital importance in Sierra Leone of social and community bonds. Such initiatives provide cause for optimism that – to draw upon the quote from Kelly (1955) that ended Chapter 6 – Sierra Leone need not be a victim of its biography but can write itself a bright new story.

## Notes

1 Even when constructs were supplied to participants in the repertory grids used in the present study, these constructs had mostly been elicited from previous groups of participants in the same setting.
2 Consider also, for example, the situation faced by the people of Afghanistan, Iraq, Syria, and Palestine, for whom conflict and oppression may be the norm.
3 For example, the ever-increasing list of diagnostic categories (some 500 in its 5th edition) contained in the *Diagnostic and Statistical Manual* of the American Psychiatric Association.
4 Government involvement was also suspected because the highest prevalence of the disease appeared to be in areas where the population tended to support the opposition party.
5 The amputee football team provided an experience of experimentation with a new role not dissimilar to Kelly's (1955) fixed-role therapy, and its 'curative factors' are also similar to those observed in group psychotherapy (Yalom, 1970), while the Community Theatre Agency may be considered to use a dramatherapy approach.

## References

Bolten, C. E. (2012) *I did it to save my life: Love and survival in Sierra Leone.* Berkeley: University of California Press.
Burgis, T. (2015) *The looting machine: Warlords, tycoons, smugglers and the systematic theft of Africa's wealth.* Glasgow: Wm Collins.
Hinzen, H., James, F. B., Sorie, J. M., Tamu, A. T. (1987) *Fishing in rivers of Sierra Leone: Oral literature.* Freetown: People's Educational Association of Sierra Leone.
Keen, D. (2005) *Conflict and collusion in Sierra Leone.* Oxford: James Currey.
Kelly, G. A. (1955) *The psychology of personal constructs.* New York: Norton. (Reprinted by Routledge, 1991)
Lilienfeld, S. O. (2007) Psychological treatments that cause harm. *Perspectives on Psychological Science,* 2: 53–70.
Maathai, W. (2009) *The challenge for Africa.* London: Heinemann.
Tschudi, F. (2016) Restorative justice. In D. A. Winter, N. Reed (Eds.), *Wiley handbook of personal construct psychology.* Chichester: Wiley-Blackwell.
Watters, E. (2010) *Crazy like us: The globalization of the American psyche.* New York: Simon and Schuster.
Winter, D. A. (1992) *Personal construct psychology in clinical practice: Theory, research and applications.* London: Routledge.
Yalom, I. D. (1970) *The theory and practice of group psychotherapy.* New York: Basic Books.

# Appendix

## Focus groups

For the first two meetings, focus group participants were asked the following: 'Tell me a story about the war you can forgive and why you can forgive it. Or, tell me a story about the war you cannot forgive and tell me why you cannot forgive it.' The participants then began a monologue that included bits of information that related to either or both of those categories.

The third focus group began by Goins saying the following:

Today I wanted us to talk some more about forgiveness, to hear some more of your opinions on what you are thinking about forgiveness. One thing that I keep hearing from different people that I talk to in Sierra Leone is, they'll say, 'I forgive but I'll never forget.' And somehow, somehow, it's, what I understand is that forgiving and forgetting, it's almost like the same thing. Can you help me to understand that?

For both groups, the question posed at the beginning of the discussion group was worded as follows:

How would you respond to *a*, or any situation from the war if there were no consequences for your actions? What if you could do whatever you wanted? What would you do if you had complete freedom to respond with no fear of punishment from the government or your parents or teacher or anyone?

From that point, children responded in various ways and Goins guided the conversation so that questions/topics such as what is listed below were covered:

What does forgiveness 'look like'?
How often do you think about the bad things that have been done to you?
What is revenge?
How do you feel about your friends who joined?
Does it help forgiveness if someone comes to you and says, 'I did wrong'?
Is it 'worse' to join the rebel forces or to be abducted?

Do you think the one who joined is guilty or the one who didn't join but was abducted is guilty?

Does the guilty one deserve forgiveness?

## Interviews

Goins made the following introductory statements to the interviewees:

- her role as a doctoral student and not being associated with any particular NGO or governmental agency
- assurance of confidentiality and that the interviewee would not be identified or identifiable
- that she would not use any information they were not comfortable with her using
- the interviewee was welcome to ask questions, make comments and request further information about her research

Questions for interviews were generally, but not strictly, as follows in the list below. This list is not comprehensive but is representative of interview questions. Modifications were made as appropriate.

What has been your experience of the war?

How do adults regard children?

When is a child no longer a child?

What is conversation like between a parent and child?

Are children seen as in need of protection?

How do you feel about the child soldiers?

How do you perceive them?

Do you want them back into the community?

How is their reintegration facilitated?

Are there rituals/cultural traditions that facilitate this?

Was the conflict a tribal one?

How is conflict reconciled within a cultural context?

Is forgiveness a relevant concept for Sierra Leoneans?

Is there a process of thought that corresponds to the word 'forgiveness'?

What is the cultural concept of that process?

What is the cultural concept of unforgiveness?

What is the cultural concept of revenge?

How does forgiveness work, what does it 'look like?'

What do you think about the government's role in promoting reintegration/ reconciliation?

What do you think about the TRC?

What do you think about the Special Court?

# Index

For Product Safety Concerns and Information please contact our EU
representative GPSR@taylorandfrancis.com
Taylor & Francis Verlag GmbH, Kaufingerstraße 24, 80331 München, Germany

www.ingramcontent.com/pod-product-compliance
Ingram Content Group UK Ltd.
Pitfield, Milton Keynes, MK11 3LW, UK
UKHW021003180425
457613UK00019B/791